It's
**OK**
to be
**NEUROTIC**

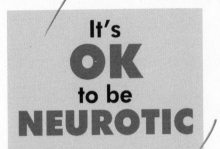

# It's
# OK
## to be
# NEUROTIC

Using Your
Neuroses to Your
Advantage

Frank Bruno, Ph.D.

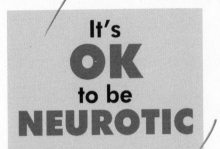

Adams Media
Avon, Massachusetts

Published by
Adams Media, an F+W Publications Company
57 Littlefield Street, Avon, MA 02322. U.S.A.
*www.adamsmedia.com*

ISBN: 1-59337-025-3

Printed in Canada

J I H G F E D C B A

**Library of Congress Cataloging-in-Publication Data**
Bruno, Frank.
It's OK to be neurotic / Frank Bruno.
p.    cm.
ISBN 1-59337-025-3
1. Neuroses--Popular works.  I. Title.
RC530.B775 2004
616.85'2—dc22
2003028019

Cover illustration by © Vicky Emptage / Getty Images.

*This book is available at quantity discounts for bulk purchases.*
*For information, call 1-800-872-5627.*

*To those who seek ways to
convert neurotic suffering into
the rewards of effective living.*

# Acknowledgments

A number of people have helped me to make *It's OK to Be Neurotic* a reality. My thanks are expressed to:

Tracy Quinn McLennan for her early recognition of the value of the book.

Danielle Chiotti, editor at Adams Media, for being a supportive and creative editor.

Eugene Brissie, my agent, for the interest he has taken in my work and for his sincere efforts on the manuscript's behalf.

Also to Sandy Smith for an excellent job of copyediting and to Laura MacLaughlin for her responsible role in supervising the final copyediting process.

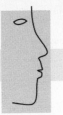

# Contents

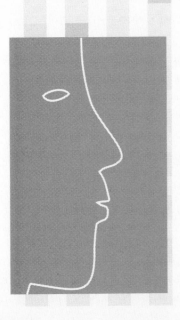

**Chapter 1**
# The Challenge of Neurosis

**You strongly suspect** that you are neurotic.

Why?

Maybe you are suffering from chronic anxiety, depression, or anger, and you recognize that your distress is essentially self-inflicted.

You may also suffer from some of the many symptoms frequently associated with a neurosis, such as phobias, obsessions, compulsions, sleep disturbances, unhealthy eating patterns, a tendency to abuse alcohol or other drugs, indecisiveness, and fatigue.

Again, you recognize—or at least suspect—that your various symptoms are also self-inflicted.

And to compound your suffering, you are sometimes angry with yourself for being neurotic. You see it as a shameful affliction—one you are loath to admit to others.

Take heart.

You're in good company. Freud, the father of psychoanalysis was—by his own admission—neurotic (see Chapter 12). I have just finished reading both the personal memoirs and a biography of General Ulysses S. Grant, commander in chief of the Union Army during the Civil War and a U.S. president. It is clear from the memoirs that Grant was neurotic. He fought a long battle with alcoholism, and he found it next to impossible to enjoy his fame and prestige. Nonetheless, he was a highly effective and successful person. Many of the world's greatest scientists, authors, composers, and artists have been neurotic. In fact, creativity and neurosis often go hand in hand.

You may have gotten the unfortunate idea that you are neurotic and that no one else is; that you're not OK, and that everyone else *is* OK. Nothing could be further from the truth. You are *not* isolated in your neurosis. It has been estimated that as many as 10 percent of adults in the United States suffer from mild to severe neurotic conditions. This translates into approximately 20 million people!

Does that number seem too high? It isn't. If anything, it is conservative. Consider that over 50 million prescriptions are written annually for antianxiety agents such as Valium and Xanax and for antidepressant agents such as Prozac and Paxil. If you happen to be neurotic, you are far from alone.

My aim in this book is not to cure you of your neurosis. No, as its title indicates, one of my aims is to convince you that you are OK just as you are, neurosis and all. Another goal is to provide guidelines for living *with* your neurosis. As the title of Chapter 6 indicates, you may have a neurosis, but it doesn't have to have you. There are ways—effective ways (without drugs!)—that can help you live happily with your neurotic self.

*It's OK to Be Neurotic* will provide you with information and the practical tips to reduce the emotional pain that may be causing you to doubt your capacity to cope with life.

## My Own Story

I confess that I, too, am neurotic. It's not a very painful admission for me anymore, because I first recognized the presence of my own neurosis when I was eighteen years old. I suffered from chronic anxiety. I still have a tendency to worry excessively, but I have learned to cope with this tendency and to minimize its effect on me and my life.

I used to abuse food, and I weighed 245 pounds when I was twenty years old. (This meant that I was about 70 pounds overweight for my height and frame.) Also, I had a strong tendency to procrastinate, and I found it difficult to finish the work I needed to in order to reach some important goals. I might also have been described as somewhat lazy. But that's only a description. *Why* was I lazy? It was because of a tendency to avoid responsibilities and important challenges, and this tendency arose from an underlying neurosis.

I majored in psychology and turned my life around. I lost weight, and I worked hard to achieve many of my goals. My story could be called "How I turned a 245-pound slob into a 175-pound man of action."

I have a Ph.D. in psychology, and I have taught the subject at the college level for more than thirty years. I have also had experience as a psychotherapist. My long and steady interest in helping others has culminated in a series of books; these include *Think Yourself Thin*, *Stop Worrying*, *Stop Procrastinating*, *The Family Mental Health Encyclopedia*, and *Psychological Symptoms*.

Everything I have learned from coping with my own neurosis and working with the neurotic problems of others is presented to you in these pages in a straightforward, easy-to-understand, and—above all else—*useful* manner.

## How This Book Is Organized

*It's OK to Be Neurotic* follows a logical, step-by-step plan, one that will help you see that you are basically OK just the way you are. You will also find ways both to cope with your neurotic tendencies and to put them to work to actually improve your life.

In each chapter, I'll discuss an aspect of neurosis in order to give you greater insight into your deeper self and the relationship of that self to the practical side of life. Toward the end of the chapter, you will find a box with a self-directed psychological "Master Strategy" with an accompanying discussion. You will find a total of twenty such strategies in the book. You can use these strategies to live more effectively with your neurotic tendencies.

How do the strategies work? I chose the word *strategy* to suggest that you can work both around and with a neurosis. You don't need to be its victim.

Let's say that you are in a small sailboat, all alone on a lake, and you are being buffeted by a high wind. If you don't know how to operate the craft's controls, you will capsize and sink. However, if you are an experienced hand, you can turn the wind to your advantage and head speedily toward your destination.

A neurosis is like the high wind. In this case, a strong force is working inside of you. You can let it sink you. Or you can learn to turn it to your advantage. The strategies in this book will enable you to turn a neurosis into something that will improve, instead of destroy, your life.

## Ten Important Things This Book Can Do for You

I want to stress again that above all this is a *useful* book, one that you can directly apply to everyday life. Here are ten important and highly specific things this book can do for you:

1. *It's OK to Be Neurotic can help you to* accept yourself, *to recognize that being neurotic is neither an unusual nor an awful affliction.* It is common for people to be neurotic. The trick is to learn a *better way* to be neurotic so you can minimize your suffering and maximize some of the advantages that can flow from having a neurotic personality.

2. *It will teach you the difference between neurosis and psychosis.* A *neurosis,* as you will learn in more detail, is a kind of chronic suffering often linked to high intelligence, imagination, and creativity. The word *psychosis,* on the other hand, refers to being out of your mind. The most common kind of functional psychosis in the United States, often treated with psychiatric drugs, is *schizophrenia,* a severe delusional disorder. In everyday language, being psychotic is referred to as "crazy," "nuts," or "out of your mind." Nope, you're not nuts because you're neurotic. You're troubled, but definitely sane.

3. *It will help you recognize that having a neurotic personality is largely something outside your immediate control*—like having blue eyes or being tall (or short). You *can,* of course, use your will and intelligence to control *how* you deal with your neurosis. But you will see that you shouldn't dump on yourself just for being neurotic.

4. *The book can make you feel better by making you aware of the positive side of neurosis.* Being neurotic is not all bad, not by any means. You will discover certain advantages that you actually have over so-called normal people. For example, as already indicated, neurotic people are often more creative than people in general. This book will demonstrate how to take advantage of your neurotic tendencies.

5. *It can help you avoid inflicting any negative aspects of your neurotic self on your loved ones.* Many a marriage or parent-child relationship has been badly damaged because of run-away neurotic tendencies, tendencies that can be expressed in unfortunate actions such as turning away love and using others as a scapegoat for aggressions.

6. *It can help you see life from a larger perspective.* The book allows you to see your existence from a more objective, scientific viewpoint. This wider viewpoint will make you feel that you are much more than a pawn of fate. Instead, you will become intensely aware of the power of your own will over the affairs in your life.

7. *It will demonstrate that you don't have to put your head down and play the social role of Victim.* (Playing the role of Victim is different from being an actual victim. Playing a role is something you do to yourself. Being an actual victim results from something adverse that happens to you.) You don't have to accept either abuse from others or the abuse that people often inflict on themselves.

8. *It will improve your self-esteem.* By seeing yourself as OK instead of as defective, you will be able to overcome the inferiority feelings associated with your neurotic tendencies.

9. *It will help you develop greater courage to cope with the challenges and difficulties of your life.* It is easy to become demoralized and feel helpless. The insights and strategies presented in the following pages will assist you in becoming a more competent, effective person.

10. It's OK to Be Neurotic *will provide you with a set of powerful tools designed to help you understand both yourself and your relation to life.* These tools are in the form of *psychological concepts.* A given psychological concept can usually be identified with a key term such as *unconscious mental life, ego defense*

*mechanism, reinforcement,* and so forth. Once you grasp these concepts and key terms, you will have a powerful language for describing and understanding both your own behavior and the behavior of others.

---

**MASTER STRATEGY 1**

### Recognize that it really is OK to be neurotic.

Starting right now, you should adopt the viewpoint that a neurosis is a challenge, not an affliction. Make the decision to see a neurosis as a way of being in the world, a way of being that is shared by as many as 20 million adults (or even more) in the United States. Appreciate the fact that being neurotic is a problem with two sides, both a downside and an upside. Both sides will be explored in this book, and your enhanced self-understanding will help you greatly improve the quality of your life.

---

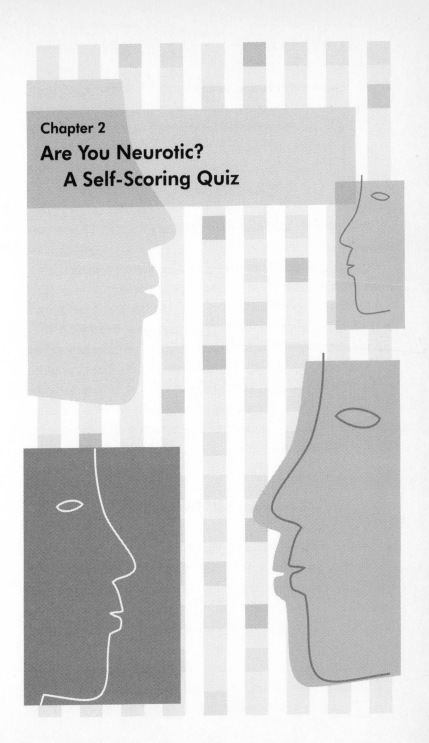

Chapter 2
## Are You Neurotic?
## A Self-Scoring Quiz

**Well, what do you think** after reading Chapter 1? Are you neurotic?

If you are absolutely sure that you're not, then there's probably not much point in reading this book.

On the other hand, if you are, this book can be a psychological lifesaver. In the next section, you will find a self-scoring quiz that will help you evaluate your present level of neurotic activity. (In both the first chapter and in this chapter, the word *neurotic* should be understood with whatever commonsense meaning it presently has for you. A formal definition with a full explanation of the concept of neurosis will follow in Chapter 3.)

## A Neurosis Self-Scoring Quiz

Answer each of the following questions *Strongly Agree, Agree, Can't Say, Disagree,* or *Strongly Disagree* by making a circle around, or a check mark next to, your choice. As is usual with psychological tests, there are no right or wrong answers. Nonetheless, your answers do reveal neurotic versus nonneurotic behavioral activity.

A scoring key with explanations follows the quiz.

There is nothing tricky or hard to understand about this quiz. The more you agree with the items, the more you are aware of neurotic tendencies that can affect the general quality of your life. Think of taking the test, and subsequently scoring it, as looking in a mirror without your clothes on. This is something that most of us have done in private in order to study our flaws. This test works in somewhat the same way. Consequently, it is essential to be honest with yourself as you answer each item. Remember, the results of this test are for your eyes and your eyes alone. Think of this test (and this book) as instruments that you can use to live more effectively, and at greater peace, with your neurosis.

1. I seem to worry about almost anything and everything.
   Strongly Agree    Agree    Can't Say    Disagree    Strongly Disagree

2. I have a hard time enjoying life.
   Strongly Agree    Agree    Can't Say    Disagree    Strongly Disagree

3. I think I have a sleep disturbance.
   Strongly Agree    Agree    Can't Say    Disagree    Strongly Disagree

4. I turn to food too often when I'm nervous or depressed.
   Strongly Agree    Agree    Can't Say    Disagree    Strongly Disagree

5. I have one or more phobias (i.e., irrational fears).
   Strongly Agree    Agree    Can't Say    Disagree    Strongly Disagree

6. I'm a perfectionist.
   Strongly Agree    Agree    Can't Say    Disagree    Strongly Disagree

7. I suffer from chronic guilt feelings, and am plagued with the idea that I've let others down.
   Strongly Agree    Agree    Can't Say    Disagree    Strongly Disagree

8. I'm overly responsible.
   Strongly Agree    Agree    Can't Say    Disagree    Strongly Disagree

9. I'm overly self-critical.

Strongly Agree     Agree     Can't Say     Disagree     Strongly Disagree

10. It seems to me that I'm almost always angry about something.

Strongly Agree     Agree     Can't Say     Disagree     Strongly Disagree

11. I have the feeling that if something can go wrong it will.

Strongly Agree     Agree     Can't Say     Disagree     Strongly Disagree

12. Life seems to be a great, overly heavy burden.

Strongly Agree     Agree     Can't Say     Disagree     Strongly Disagree

13. I don't honestly know if I can say that I either like or love myself.

Strongly Agree     Agree     Can't Say     Disagree     Strongly Disagree

14. I regularly use cigarettes, alcohol, or drugs to tranquilize myself.

Strongly Agree     Agree     Can't Say     Disagree     Strongly Disagree

15. The faults in other people are both obvious and irritating.

Strongly Agree     Agree     Can't Say     Disagree     Strongly Disagree

16. I have compulsions—magical rituals that help me cope.

Strongly Agree     Agree     Can't Say     Disagree     Strongly Disagree

17. I frequently feel that nobody really understands me.

Strongly Agree     Agree     Can't Say     Disagree     Strongly Disagree

18. I could probably do great things, but something seems to be standing in my way.

Strongly Agree     Agree     Can't Say     Disagree     Strongly Disagree

19. I feel low with the blues or the "blahs" much of the time.

Strongly Agree     Agree     Can't Say     Disagree     Strongly Disagree

20. I'm frequently tired and lack energy. And I suspect that this is due to my emotional state, not my physical health.

Strongly Agree     Agree     Can't Say     Disagree     Strongly Disagree

21. It seems to me that my heart pounds heavily more often than it should.
    Strongly Agree     Agree     Can't Say     Disagree     Strongly Disagree

22. I don't like to go outside of my house by myself.
    Strongly Agree     Agree     Can't Say     Disagree     Strongly Disagree

23. The presence of insects makes me tense and uncomfortable.
    Strongly Agree     Agree     Can't Say     Disagree     Strongly Disagree

24. I don't much like to go to parties and meet new people.
    Strongly Agree     Agree     Can't Say     Disagree     Strongly Disagree

25. I am more or less a mystery to myself.
    Strongly Agree     Agree     Can't Say     Disagree     Strongly Disagree

26. I suffer quite a bit from constipation.
    Strongly Agree     Agree     Can't Say     Disagree     Strongly Disagree

27. I feel quite upset if I forget to take my daily vitamin pills.
    Strongly Agree     Agree     Can't Say     Disagree     Strongly Disagree

28. Although other people treat me as if I'm beautiful (or handsome), I don't think so at all. In fact, sometimes I feel that my face or body is kind of ugly.
    Strongly Agree     Agree     Can't Say     Disagree     Strongly Disagree

29. Most of the time I think of other people as superior to me in some way.
    Strongly Agree     Agree     Can't Say     Disagree     Strongly Disagree

30. I can't stand snakes.
    Strongly Agree     Agree     Can't Say     Disagree     Strongly Disagree

31. My dreams often have a fantastic quality, tending to be about people and places far removed from my daily experiences.
    Strongly Agree     Agree     Can't Say     Disagree     Strongly Disagree

32. I am prone to have headaches induced by tension or stressful experiences.

Strongly Agree    Agree    Can't Say    Disagree    Strongly Disagree

33. Sometimes I think I'm allergic to almost everything.

Strongly Agree    Agree    Can't Say    Disagree    Strongly Disagree

34. I'm a picky eater. Only a fairly restricted set of foods appeal to me.

Strongly Agree    Agree    Can't Say    Disagree    Strongly Disagree

35. I have to double-check and triple-check almost everything I do.

Strongly Agree    Agree    Can't Say    Disagree    Strongly Disagree

36. I find it very hard to control my tendency to magnify my problems.

Strongly Agree    Agree    Can't Say    Disagree    Strongly Disagree

37. I know it's silly, but I feel as if everyone I know has to like me.

Strongly Agree    Agree    Can't Say    Disagree    Strongly Disagree

38. I suffer a lot from what seems to be muscle pain, but I don't know if there's any physical basis for it.

Strongly Agree    Agree    Can't Say    Disagree    Strongly Disagree

39. I have a disturbing, overactive imagination.

Strongly Agree    Agree    Can't Say    Disagree    Strongly Disagree

40. It's just awful when things don't go the way I want them to go.

Strongly Agree    Agree    Can't Say    Disagree    Strongly Disagree

41. I have a tendency to bite my nails, chew on my fingertips, or otherwise pick on my body.

Strongly Agree    Agree    Can't Say    Disagree    Strongly Disagree

42. I kid myself a lot.

Strongly Agree    Agree    Can't Say    Disagree    Strongly Disagree

43. I find it very hard to relax.

Strongly Agree     Agree     Can't Say     Disagree     Strongly Disagree

44. I don't seem to get enough pleasure out of life.

Strongly Agree     Agree     Can't Say     Disagree     Strongly Disagree

45. Sometimes I feel that I would just like to live on mood-modifying drugs.

Strongly Agree     Agree     Can't Say     Disagree     Strongly Disagree

46. My sex life leaves a lot to be desired.

Strongly Agree     Agree     Can't Say     Disagree     Strongly Disagree

47. There's a lot to be said for the statement, "Life is a tale full of sound and fury, told by an idiot, signifying nothing."

Strongly Agree     Agree     Can't Say     Disagree     Strongly Disagree

48. I often feel restless and edgy.

Strongly Agree     Agree     Can't Say     Disagree     Strongly Disagree

49. I tend to minimize my accomplishments and abilities.

Strongly Agree     Agree     Can't Say     Disagree     Strongly Disagree

50. My general energy level is much too low.

Strongly Agree     Agree     Can't Say     Disagree     Strongly Disagree

## Self-Scoring Answer Key

Before you score the quiz, I need to make a couple of important points. First, this quiz is informal and does not meet the criteria of a standardized psychological test. Such tests have, on the basis of a substantial amount of data and research, demonstrated themselves to be both valid and reliable. (A *valid* test measures what it is supposed to measure. A *reliable* test gives stable, repeatable measurements.) Standardized tests are used by clinical psychologists and psychiatrists to make formal diagnoses. An informal test like the one you have just taken is indicative (that is, may indicate some tendencies), but not diagnostic. In brief, don't use the test as the basis for a self-diagnosis of any kind.

Second, the approach of this book—that it's OK to be neurotic—means that any score you obtain represents not psychological sickness, but a challenge to your ability to adjust and adapt to life. Consequently, think of the score as a kind of taking of your neurosis temperature. A high temperature can go down. It's not a permanent fixture of your life. Similarly, if you have many signs and symptoms of a neurosis, there is no reason that these signs and symptoms may not become milder with time and self-directed psychological work. Use the quiz to evaluate how you are doing right now; then take it again a month or two from now after you have read the book and have applied some of its suggestions.

Although it *is* OK to be neurotic, it's not OK to let the signs and symptoms of neurosis—as indicated by the quiz items—overwhelm you and interfere with the quality of your life.

In order to score the test, give yourself 4 points for every Strongly Agree answer, 3 points for every Agree answer, 2 points for every Can't Say answer, 1 point for every Disagree answer, and 0 points for every Strongly Disagree answer. The highest obtainable score is 200. The lowest obtainable score is zero.

If your score is 200–167, the signs and symptoms of a neurosis appear to be highly evident. It is quite likely that you are allowing your neurotic tendencies to have too strong an influence on your life. Your neurosis temperature is very hot, and you should seek ways to bring it down.

If your score is 166–134, the signs and symptoms of a neurosis are certainly present, but your neurotic tendencies are tempered to some extent. Your neurosis temperature is still fairly hot, but it appears that you have some degree of control over your impulses.

If your score is 133–101, the signs and symptoms of a neurosis are there, but your neurotic tendencies are highly modulated. With scores in this range, it appears that your efforts to manage your neurosis are meeting with some success.

A score of 100 or less suggests that you are near or below the median for this type of test, and that your signs and symptoms fall within an average zone.

If your score is on the high side, don't be overly discouraged. You don't have to be at the mercy of your neurotic tendencies. That's what this book is for—to provide you with a set of practical ways to manage your neurosis. There are two aspects to this. First, you can use the book to minimize any suffering associated with your neurosis. Second, you can use it to maximize the positive aspects of being neurotic.

### MASTER STRATEGY 2

## Work to lower your neurosis temperature.

Even if your neurosis temperature is high now, it can go down. Like a body temperature, a psychological temperature is a variable thing. It is not a permanent fact about you, but something that is subject to change. In this attitude, you'll find hope for change.

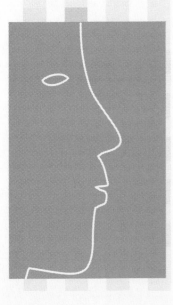

# Chapter 3
# What Is a Neurosis Anyway?:
## Key Questions and Answers

**It's easy to say,** "Jake is obviously neurotic. He worries all the time."

It is equally easy to say, "Alice is hopelessly neurotic. She's such a perfectionist."

Is the word *neurosis* overused? Does the word now cover so much territory that it is nearly meaningless? There is a risk that this can happen when we write and talk about neurosis. So the time has come to sharpen our understanding. Let's attempt to answer the question, "What is a neurosis anyway?"

Here is a core definition: *A neurosis exists in an individual if that individual suffers chronic anxiety out of proportion to realistic threats.* That's it in a nutshell. There's more—a lot more—to be said. But the core definition will be helpful. It's central. Everything else in this chapter revolves around it.

Before going further, consider a few key words in this definition. A neurosis causes *chronic* anxiety; that is, it is something that recurs at least on occasion and does not merely affect you once or twice. Also, a neurosis causes distress that is out of proportion to your actual situation. If you are in the middle of an earthquake and you experience fear, that is not the sign of a neurosis; that's just good sense.

## The Origin of the Idea

The word *neurosis* is related to such words as *nerves* and *neurology*. Neurologists study and treat nerve disorders. This explains why in the early days of psychotherapy so many psychiatrists and psychotherapists were also neurologists. Freud was trained in neurology. So was Viktor Frankl, the great existential therapist.

Originally, a neurosis was thought to be a weakness of the nerves, and people searched for a physical basis for such conditions. As long ago as 400 B.C., Hippocrates, the father of Western medicine, believed that hysteria was caused by a "wandering" uterus. (The Greek word for uterus is *hyster*.) Hysteria is a kind of neurosis characterized by false symptoms with no real neurological cause. For example, an individual may imagine that he or she cannot move a limb, and the belief that that arm or leg can't be moved becomes a self-fulfilling prophecy. The person is for all intents and purposes paralyzed.

Freud recognized that hysteria is essentially a psychological condition caused by emotional conflict, and not a problem with the position of the uterus. One of Freud's older colleagues mocked him by saying, "But my dear Dr. Freud. Are you a fool or what? Men do not have a uterus. How can they, consequently, suffer from hysteria?" Freud has been proved to be correct; men can and do suffer from hysteria and, of course, don't have a uterus. Today, however, *hysteria* is thought of as an antiquated term. Current psychiatric language replaces hysteria with the term *conversion disorder*, suggesting that in this kind of neurosis, anxiety has been converted into a bodily symptom.

The first book concerning psychoanalysis was *Studies in Hysteria* by Josef Breuer and Sigmund Freud, published in

1895. So you can see that the concept of neurosis has a long history of association with pathology (a sickness of the mind or the body).

This book recognizes the pathological side of neurosis, but, as you will see, it also develops the positive side of neurosis. We will explore how neurotic energy can be turned to your advantage, how it can be used *for* you instead of against you.

In order to sharpen your overall understanding of the concept of neurosis, the balance of this chapter asks and answers questions about the meaning and varieties of neurosis.

## HOW DOES A NEUROSIS DIFFER FROM A PSYCHOSIS?

It is not uncommon for neurotic people to be thought of as "crazy" or "nuts." This is unfortunate. It is true that neurotic people usually have significant problems in living, that they experience emotional turmoil, that they do worry a lot, and that they are often eccentric. Nonetheless, all of this is far, far away from real madness.

There *is* a condition called psychosis, but it is not the same as neurosis. A psychosis exists when a person is out of touch with reality. He or she experiences a severe thought disorder characterized by delusions. Delusions are false beliefs. For example, Rowena, a thirty-three-year-old mother of three daughters, believes that she is a queen of Mars. She is living on Earth in temporary exile, and her three daughters will become princesses of the red planet someday when John Carter teleports her and her children back home. (John Carter is a fictional hero who had adventures on Mars. Edgar Rice Burroughs, the author of *Tarzan of the Apes,* created Carter.)

Neurotic people tend not to be delusional. Their struggle, on the whole, is with the here and the now—with the challenges and frustrations of everyday life. Neurosis and psychosis are two very different kinds of conditions.

A psychosis can be functional or organic. The most common kind of functional psychosis in the United States is *schizophrenia*. Again, like psychosis in general, schizophrenia is a severe thought disorder characterized by delusions. It is called "functional" because its organic basis is difficult to specify. Nonetheless, there is compelling evidence that genetic factors do in fact play a role in the disorder.

An organic psychosis is one that is caused by an actual breakdown in the integrity of the nervous system. Infections or injuries that damage the brain are principal causes of organic psychoses.

None of the severe pathology mentioned should be confused with a neurosis. A neurosis is a far, far milder condition—something you can learn to live with.

## How does a neurosis differ from a personality disorder?

Although a neurosis and a personality disorder are both behavioral disorders, they exhibit important differences. As already noted, the core of a neurosis is *anxiety*. A person with a personality disorder, on the other hand, will often experience little or no anxiety. A *personality disorder* is characterized by warped or exaggerated traits. A *trait*, in psychological theory, is a stable disposition to act in a particular way. For example, if Nancy studies regularly two hours a week for every hour she attends college class, she might be said to possess the trait of *studiousness*. (No, studying like

23

this is not a disorder; it's not pathological. It's just an example of a trait.)

One type of personality disorder that provides a distinct contrast to a neurosis is an *antisocial personality disorder*. The term does not mean that the individual is a hermit or reclusive. On the contrary, persons with this disorder are often charming and superficially friendly. An antisocial personality disorder is characterized by a lack of conscience and a tendency to manipulate others. Persons with this disorder can use and abuse others without suffering pangs of guilt or anxiety for their misdeeds. For example, Alfred is an unscrupulous salesperson. He peddles worthless stocks and bonds to elderly people, often ruining them financially. Alfred drives an expensive car, sleeps well, and experiences no emotional distress. (An older term for an antisocial personality disorder is *psychopath*.)

If you are neurotic, you are probably nothing like Alfred. You worry when you think you have done something even a little wrong. You experience guilt often and easily, even for small misdeeds. Your conscience, if anything, is overactive. Persons with an antisocial personality disorder are *undersocialized*. You, on the other hand, are likely to be *oversocialized*. You let others use and abuse you instead of using and abusing them.

## WHAT ARE THE KINDS OF NEUROSIS?

First of all, in modern psychiatric nomenclature the term *neurosis* is no longer used as a diagnosis. It is correct and proper to say that a person suffers from "neurotic conflict" or that "a neurotic process is present." But it is not considered quite accurate for a clinical psychologist or a psychiatrist to say, "My diagnosis is that the patient has a neurosis." This is not considered to be specific enough.

Consequently, the American Psychiatric Association's diagnostic manual identifies a set of anxiety disorders. This cluster of related disorders is more or less synonymous with what most people would call "a neurosis." These disorders include (1) generalized anxiety disorder, (2) phobic disorder, (3) obsessive-compulsive disorder (OCD), and (4) post-traumatic stress disorder (PTSD).

**Generalized anxiety disorder** is characterized by a tendency to worry too much about anything and everything. The term *free-floating anxiety* is used to describe this kind of chronic worry, because the anxiety seems to follow the individual around like a dark cloud. For example, Emma is a twenty-three-year-old college student who can worry about almost any situation that presents itself. She worries about her appearance when she goes out on a date, even though she is attractive and well dressed. She worries about failing examinations, even when she is well prepared. She worries that friends will reject her, even when they are warm and natural with her. People who suffer from a generalized anxiety disorder are among the principal candidates for drugs such as Valium and Xanax.

**Phobic disorders** are characterized by irrational fears. There are many such fears. They include fears of heights, blood, storms, high places, closed spaces, strangers, public places, and more. These fears have specific names, some of which are commonly known. For example, a fear of closed spaces is called *claustrophobia*.

**Obsessive-compulsive disorder** (OCD) is characterized by magical rituals that reduce the anxiety arising from odd or irrational ideas. For example, the famous inventor Nikola Tesla was obsessed with the "danger" from germs on his plates, utensils, and glasses. A lifelong bachelor, he ate in the dining room of fine hotels. In some cases he requested as many as twenty-one fresh white napkins so he could carefully wipe the plates and other items. He clearly recognized that his own behavior was neurotic. As a trained scientist, he knew that the ritual wiping would do nothing to eliminate germs. The behavior was in essence magical.

In spite of his many hang-ups, Tesla was highly creative and made many scientific contributions. For example, he was the first engineer to demonstrate the practical aspects of alternating electrical current. And, despite all of those germs he worried about, he lived to be eighty-seven years old.

**Post-traumatic stress disorder** (PTSD) is characterized by anxiety arising from surviving a highly painful or dangerous experience. Examples of such experiences include floods, earthquakes, fires, military combat, and rape. Not only anxiety, but also depression and sleep disturbances go along with PTSD.

Although, as indicated, a neurosis is not a specific disorder, it is still meaningful to speak of "being neurotic." A neurotic person is one who suffers from an anxiety disorder. A neurotic person approaches life with what the existential philosopher Søren Kierkegaard called "fear and trembling." A neurotic person is a sensitive individual who is highly aware of the dangers—both physical and emotional—of being alive.

## WHAT CAUSES SOMEONE TO
## SUFFER FROM A NEUROSIS?

There are various viewpoints used to explain the existence of a neurosis in an individual. The principal ones are (1) psychoanalytic, (2) behavioral, (3) biological, (4) cognitive, and (5) existential.

The **psychoanalytic** point of view states that a neurosis arises because of inner emotional conflict. The viewpoint was first proposed by Sigmund Freud, the father of psychoanalysis. Freud asserted that there are three parts to the personality: the id, the ego, and the superego. The *id* is the primal self. It is inborn and oriented toward pleasure. The *ego* is the conscious self. It is born out of the id because of the necessity to cope with the frustrations and challenges of the world. Consequently, the ego is oriented toward reality. The *superego* is the moral self. It is the reflection of the teachings of our parents and other authority figures.

According to the psychoanalytic viewpoint, anxiety arises when the individual senses that the impulses of the id are at odds with the moral prescriptions of the superego. For example, Gabrielle, a married woman, finds her brother-in-law very attractive. Her id says, "Go and have some great sex with this guy." Her superego says, "You're disgusting. You have to be true to your husband. You took vows and promised to be faithful." She fears that she will actually act on her id impulses and cheat on her husband with his brother. She hasn't done so yet, but nonetheless the possibility exists. The threat is associated with the possibility that she won't be able to control her own impulses. Her ego, being reality oriented, keeps her from doing anything foolish.

According to this viewpoint, one way to look at neurosis

is as an ongoing conflict between the forbidden impulses of the id and the moral code of the superego.

Persons with a strong, reality-oriented ego are unlikely to make fools out of themselves. People who live life realistically are not dominated by their forbidden id impulses. Ernest Jones, a psychoanalyst and Freud's principal biographer, said, "The art of living is the art of compromise." The person who finds a way to live with a neurosis discovers a middle road between the forbidden impulses of the id and the strict dictates of the superego.

The **behavioral** viewpoint suggests that a neurosis arises because of maladaptive learning. In essence, a neurosis is a set of bad habits. These can be bad emotional habits or bad action habits. Here is an example of a bad emotional habit. When Kaitlin was five years old she was sexually molested by a freckle-faced, red-haired sixteen-year-old male babysitter. Now twenty-two years old, Kaitlin can't stand red-haired men. The sight of one makes her flesh crawl. She has forgotten that she was molested. All that remains is the strange, seemingly meaningless, aversion to men with red hair. Neurotic aversions of all kinds may be explained in terms of associations with bad experiences in the past. The great Russian physiologist Ivan Pavlov called these kinds of reactions *conditioned reflexes,* suggesting that they were acquired by experience, that they were learned, and that they were not inborn like natural, or unconditioned, reflexes.

Here is an example of a bad action habit. When Dalton was in grammar school, he found it difficult to learn how to do arithmetic. In high school he earned a D in algebra. Now, a college student interested in majoring in psychology, he avoids taking the required statistics course because he doesn't believe he can pass it. Dalton is twenty-five years old, a veteran with an honorable discharge, and probably quite able to pass the statistics course. Nonetheless, he suffers from *learned helplessness,* a condition associated with his past failures. He mistakenly generalizes from the past, thinking that he's the same person he was when he was a child. We can suffer from learned helplessness in almost any area of our lives that demands we be competent. Learned helplessness often contributes to neurotic anxiety. You can easily imagine that if Dalton decides to sign up for the statistics course that he will be tense and nervous, that he will fear failure. *Avoidance,* shown by not taking the required course, is the bad action habit associated with learned helplessness.

The **biological** viewpoint asserts that a neurosis has an organic basis. One possibility is that a tendency to be neurotic is inherited, that it has a genetic basis. Indeed, there seems to be evidence in favor of this idea. A trait known as *neuroticism,* a tendency to suffer from chronic anxiety and its related symptoms, does seem to be a given of some personalities, and this trait may be evident to some extent even at the pre-school level of development.

A second possibility is that neurotic symptoms are caused by imbalances in brain chemistry. Certain key *neurotransmitters,* chemical messengers in the brain, may be in short supply. The drug Prozac raises the levels of one of these neurotransmitters, serotonin.

A third possibility is that a condition called *hypoglycemia,* or low blood sugar, can induce or aggravate anxiety and depression. The biological viewpoint asserts that there is no formal, rigid distinction between the organic level and the psychological level of explanation.

The **cognitive** viewpoint asserts that neurosis is due to thinking incorrectly about the world, including the social world of other people. One of the principal founding figures associated with this viewpoint, Albert Ellis, states that irrational ideas induce adverse emotional states. For example, Ilene has been asked to give an oral book report in an English literature class. She thinks, "I'll get confused and I'll make a fool out of myself. I'll just die if the class laughs at me." These and similar self-directed thoughts will generate extreme anxiety. The idea that she will die *is* irrational because Ilene will not literally die and become a corpse if she is laughed at. Nonetheless, at an emotional level she feels as threatened as if a gun were pointed at her.

The cognitive viewpoint recognizes that irrational ideas must come from somewhere. They sprout and flower from psychological seeds planted in past experiences. Both the psychoanalytic and behavioral viewpoints stress the important role that learning and adverse experience play in neurotic conditions. Ilene was made to feel stupid by an authoritarian father. She is shy and doubtful, and her conscious ideas about herself reflect these emotional attitudes.

The **existential** viewpoint holds that anxiety is part and parcel of the human condition. If you are aware, conscious, and perceive clearly the risks and threats of life, it is almost impossible to avoid unwanted anxiety. As earlier noted, the existential philosopher Kierkegaard used the phrase *fear and trembling* to describe the human condition. It is natural to have an alarm reaction in response to much of what life presents. The effective person knows when to listen to an alarm and to take it seriously. He or she also knows how to recognize a false alarm. The art of recognizing false alarms greatly reduces anxiety and improves the individual's ability to function in the everyday world.

Which viewpoint should you accept? The correct answer is, "All of them!" They all make sense. They all account for some portion of neurotic behavior. Understanding the viewpoints and discovering ways to apply them to daily living will make it possible for you to become more and more OK with your own neurosis.

## DOES BEING NEUROTIC MEAN YOU HAVE TO LIVE A LIFE OF MISERY AND SUFFERING?

The answer to this question is quite definitely "No."

Freud was once asked, "What is the purpose of psychoanalysis?" He answered, "To replace neurotic suffering with ordinary human misery." His answer is amusing and sad at the same time, and it may seem that he is not being completely serious. However, taking his answer at face value, Freud seems to be saying that life inevitably contains a certain amount of emotional pain and suffering. This is, as existential philosophy asserts, the human condition. However, neither you nor I need to aggravate ordinary suffering by magnifying it through the lens of a neurotic personality. We can learn to put, so to speak, our neurotic vision of the world to one side and look at life plainly and realistically. Then we will be free from unnecessary suffering.

Being neurotic would seem to doom a person to a life of misery and suffering. But being neurotic does *not* have to poison your existence. It is extremely difficult to completely rid yourself of a neurosis through psychotherapy, drug therapy, or self-directed interventions. However, it is possible to *manage* a neurotic condition, manage it in such a way that the effects of a neurosis are negligible. By now I hope you're aware that the aim of this book is to show you how such self-management is possible.

## HOW DOES THE STRATEGIC APPROACH TO SELF-MANAGEMENT WORK?

According to my dictionary, one definition of a strategy is *a plan or technique for achieving some end.* Let's say that you're short on cash this month. A survival strategy might be to eat beans and day-old bread until your next paycheck. Let's say that it's snowing and you want to go home from work. A practical strategy might be to drive slowly on good roads. You find a way to eat and a way to go home even though you're short on cash or it's snowing. In other words, an adverse circumstance doesn't have to get you down or stop you if you have a practical strategy.

In the same way, having a neurosis doesn't have to get you down or stop you if you use practical self-directed strategies to get around the neurosis. That is the method of this book.

---

### MASTER STRATEGY 3

### *Adopt the positive attitude that a neurosis is not an affliction, but a challenge.*

No doubt about it—being neurotic has its downside. Nonetheless, being neurotic also has its upside. Neurotic people tend to be sensitive, intelligent, reflective, and creative. You should be thankful that you have these traits. You can allow these traits, no matter how desirable they may seem, to wound you if you don't know how to manage them. On the other hand, by employing the self-directed strategies described in this book, you will learn how to turn your neurotic disposition into an advantage.

---

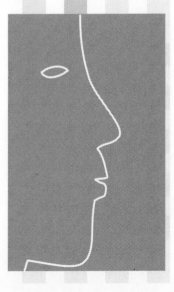

# Chapter 4
# The Disadvantages of
## Being Neurotic

**The disadvantages of** being neurotic are transparent. If you are like most neurotic people, you already know you are prone to chronic worry, depression, or anger. You feel emotionally vulnerable. Sometimes you feel like a cork tossed on a stormy emotional ocean.

Just review most of the statements you agreed with on the self-scoring quiz in Chapter 2. This is your personal list of the disadvantages of being neurotic.

This chapter would be of no use to you if it just described the disadvantages of being neurotic. That would just drag you down some more. On the contrary, the purpose of the chapter is to show you ways to cope with these disadvantages, and even sometimes turn them into advantages. And in the following chapter, we'll even consider how to maximize the positive aspects of having a neurosis. (Yes, there are some.)

The philosopher Friedrich Nietzsche wrote, "That which does not destroy me strengthens me." The effort you make to overcome and manage neurosis can turn you into a stronger person, better able to deal with whatever life has to offer.

## Common Neurotic Disadvantages

Let's be specific. In the first half of this chapter, I'll target the disadvantages of being neurotic that are of particular importance.

But don't worry: In the second half of the chapter, we'll take them up one by one and show you ways to cope effectively with these downsides to neurosis.

## Fatigue

Neurotic people often complain of being fatigued. Camilla G. is the thirty-four-year-old mother of three boys. She is a full-time homemaker and feels overwhelmed by her responsibilities. In a counseling session with me, she said, "I feel tired all the time. I've complained to doctors, but they say there's nothing wrong. How can I feel so darn tired and not be sick somehow?"

I told her, "Fatigue is a symptom. It can, of course, be a symptom of a physical illness. But it can also be a psychological symptom. If you feel overloaded, this induces stress. A human being in a state of almost constant stress will feel fatigued."

The pioneer stress researcher Hans Selye clearly showed the ways that stress takes a heavy toll on both the mind and the body.

## Shyness

Often lacking deep self-confidence, neurotic people are frequently shy. They feel they are being scrutinized and judged by others. Sherman V., a forty-one-year-old mechanical engineer, told me, "I feel as if I'm living in a fishbowl. I think that people are examining me and finding me too skinny and sort of slow-witted. I hate it when my supervisor looks at my work. Even if he doesn't say anything openly critical, I think he's nitpicking in his mind."

John Steinbeck wrote such books as *Of Mice and Men* and *The Grapes of Wrath* and was awarded a Nobel Prize in literature. You would think that he must have been a highly effective and self-confident adult. Yet he suffered from shyness as a child. His biographer, Thomas Kiernan, says that at age three Steinbeck's face had a rodentlike aspect and his ears jutted out from his head at a sharp angle. His mother called him "my little squirrel." His older sisters called him "muskrat" and "mouse." The seeds of shyness, planted in early childhood, sprouted and plagued Steinbeck for many years.

A distinction can be made between *situational* shyness and *chronic* shyness. Almost all people experience shyness in certain situations. Examples include a job interview or having to socialize with people of a higher social status. Chronic shyness, on the other hand, is characterized by a tendency to be shy in almost all situations. It is an ongoing steady-state kind of personal misery. This is the type of shyness associated with neurosis.

### Perfectionism

One undesirable trait often associated with neurosis is a tendency to demand perfection. People with this trait might demand perfection of themselves or of others. They might also expect perfection in accomplishments and outcomes. Jelena H. is a twenty-four-year-old college student. She aspires to become a nurse. She says, "Since I returned to college, I have earned a straight A average. I feel that this is a must. I know I can probably get into a good nursing school with a high B average, and my friends say that's good enough. But I hate the words *good enough*. I study almost every night until two A.M. I'm getting dark circles under my eyes. My boyfriend is about to break up with me. I don't know what I'll do if and when I get a B in a course. I feel like it will plunge me into a depression."

Perfectionistic people tend to demand that their children be excessively polite, that a partner be constantly loving and understanding, that clothing always be unwrinkled and spotless, that sinks and mirrors shine, that automobiles gleam, and so forth. It is a great burden to carry.

### Being Overly Responsible

It would seem impossible to be *overly* responsible. After all, being responsible is generally regarded as a desirable trait. This is particularly true when we live in a world where irresponsibility is rampant. Psychiatrist William Glasser, author of *Reality Therapy,* equates many mental health problems with a lack of responsibility. People who don't pay their bills, who drive over the speed limit, who don't care about the feelings of others, who are seldom on time, and so forth are a problem to themselves and others.

Nonetheless, it *is* possible to be overly responsible. You can care too much. You can take life too seriously. Neurotic people are often *oversocialized,* meaning that they try too hard to walk the straight and narrow and they try too hard to keep others happy. All this effort generates anxiety: "Will they like me?" "Will he approve?" "Will I be rejected by my friend?" These kinds of questions can plague someone who feels that he or she must conform to the expectations of others at all costs.

When you are oversocialized, you try too hard to please others. You let them use you and abuse you. You feel manipulated and controlled. And this is a contributing factor to depression.

## *Irrational Thinking*

Seventeenth-century philosopher René Descartes said, "I think, therefore I am." This is one of the most often quoted remarks in history. But what exactly did Descartes mean? Why did he say it? Common sense says he must have known he existed. Actually, he wasn't doubting his existence. He was doubting the validity of what he had been taught by others, the agreed-upon knowledge of his day and age. He asked himself what he could be sure of. And he came up with the fact that he existed ("I am.").

So he then asked himself how he could be sure he existed. And he answered, "Because I am thinking." This logic resulted in his famous dictum, "I think, therefore I am."

It would appear that Descartes was engaging in some pretty rational thinking. And his dictum underscores the essential quality that thought plays in human existence.

The thoughts we think are often the immediate causes of why we act and feel as we do.

Our emotional states in particular are often induced by our thoughts.

Rita thinks, "I'm a failure as a mother." And this induces a state of depression.

Harley thinks, "Nothing ever goes right in my life." He becomes depressed as well.

Neurotic people tend to think irrational thoughts, thoughts that are not logical. This is because they are prone to make *cognitive errors*. These are thoughts that warp reality and oversimplify it. Rita is making an error called *either-or thinking*. She is thinking that she is a failure as a mother because she has just had an argument with her fourteen-year-old daughter. For the moment she does not focus on the fact that most of the time her daughter is a loving and polite person who gets good grades.

Harley is making an error called *catastrophic thinking*. He has adopted Murphy's Law: "If anything can go wrong, it will." He has temporarily forgotten about the many, many things that go right in his life. His wife is in love with him. His income is above average. His health is good.

Irrational thoughts tempt us. You do not have to be out of your mind to have irrational thoughts. They are common in people who are perfectly sane. And they are one of the serious disadvantages of being neurotic.

## How to Cope with Neurotic Disadvantages

You are not helpless in the face of neurotic disadvantages. You can disarm them. You can neutralize their adverse effects. You do not have to play the role of victim. This section presents a group of self-directed psychological strategies that will help you minimize the disadvantages of being neurotic.

### Coping with Fatigue

SEEK WAYS TO REDUCE STRESS OVERLOAD.

In the case of chronic fatigue you should, of course, first establish that your fatigue does not have a biological basis and is not primarily a medical problem. If you have an undiagnosed case of diabetes, have unsuspected high blood pressure, have a vitamin deficiency, are significantly overweight, or have a similar problem, then these possible causes of fatigue need to be addressed first.

However, you can suffer from fatigue due to stress. As was indicated earlier, if you feel overloaded, if you feel like Atlas carrying the world on your shoulders, you are bound to suffer from chronic fatigue. But what can you do? Your first reaction might be, "Well, I *am* overloaded." This may be true, but it is important to recognize that you have a realm of choice, that there are burdens you don't have to take on.

Camilla G., the mother of three boys, grew to recognize that she was trying to be a supermother. She had all of the boys enrolled in various activities outside school. She served three days a week as a teacher's aide. She tried to cook a well-balanced meal every night. She did all of the house-cleaning. She was piling work upon work on herself. Her own interests and desires were being neglected.

Over time she found ways to assign some responsibilities to her husband, and she hired a part-time housecleaner. She and her husband agreed they could afford to eat out at least one night a week at a family restaurant. Setting up a small studio in a spare room, she returned to painting in oils a few hours a week. She began to enjoy life a little more, and many of her fatigue symptoms diminished.

It is natural to feel fatigue in response to doing things we don't enjoy. It's a subconscious avoidance reaction. We all have to do things we don't want to do, but the trick is to place a limit on them. And we need to make sure that we don't forget about what we really do want to do.

### Start a low-intensity exercise program.

Moderate exercise stimulates your brain to produce *endorphins,* a word derived from "endogenous morphines." Endorphins are naturally occurring opiates in the human nervous system, and they are associated with a feeling of well-being. Riding a bicycle or going for a walk for a half-hour three times a week is sufficient to get a beneficial effect from endorphins. I use a stationery exercise bicycle almost every Monday, Wednesday, and Friday morning before I leave for the college. Contrary to what you might think, it has been found that mild exercise does not make you more tired. It gives you, overall, a lift.

## Coping with Shyness

### LIST YOUR ASSETS.

Let's face it. You won't get over chronic shyness over-night. This is because shyness is an involuntary reaction. It's outside of the control of your will. You feel shy in a situation and you think, "I just can't help it." So you need to take a step back from your shyness and look at its psycholog-ical roots. You will find that shyness is related to a kind of negative self-judgment. You *think* you feel shy because others are judging you. And shyness is a form of extreme self-consciousness. But don't you see that you are really judging yourself? You are looking at yourself in the mirror of your mind, and you see your defects. They seem very large to you, and you incorrectly believe that others are paying a lot of attention to them.

You need instead to focus on your assets. So get out a piece of paper and make a list of your good points, both physical and psychological. Identify what is good about your body. Perhaps it's your hair, your eyes, or your hands. Identify what is good about your personality. Perhaps you have a good sense of humor, are loyal, or are very nurturing. Get rid of the distortions in that mirror of your mind, and you will see yourself in a better light. It will help you feel more confident in the presence of others.

Obviously, shyness is related to an inferiority complex. We'll discuss that problem more later.

A warning: Don't try to overcome shyness by becoming brash and aggressive. It won't work. It's not the real you. And such a tactic will almost certainly backfire on you emotionally and result in even more depression and anxiety. Instead, you should recognize that a certain level of shyness is tolerable. You need to diminish the intensity of your shyness and its impact on your life. You don't have to feel obligated to remove it entirely.

### SEEK WAYS TO DRAW SOMETHING OF VALUE FROM YOUR SHYNESS.

You will recall that the author John Steinbeck was bothered by shyness for a number of years. In adolescence and young adulthood, his shyness drove him into himself. He began to write out of his loneliness and the need to find a way to express himself to others. And look where it led. He was awarded a Nobel Prize for literature.

Some shy people turn to acting as an avocation or a profession. It is a way they can use the mask of the role they are playing to diminish the intensity of their shyness. Their inner insecurity often fuels an intensity and power in their performances that is lacking in people who don't have their emotional need. Chapter 8 has a further discussion on the possible uses of neurosis in enhancing creativity.

Shyness is associated with the trait of introversion. Introverted people tend to look within themselves. They tend to see life in profound terms and to appreciate its richness. As a shy person, it is likely that you are less superficial than many other people. Your introversion is OK. We live in an extroverted culture that tends to look down on the introverted person. And your underlying shyness is OK, too. However, it is important to look for ways to minimize any adverse influence it has on your life. Simultaneously, you want to look for ways to maximize its potential for enriching your life.

## Coping with Perfectionism

### LEARN TO THINK IN TERMS OF "GOOD ENOUGH" INSTEAD OF PERFECTION.

Jelena H., the nursing student, said that she hated the words *good enough*. And yet it was this very set of words that she decided to learn to accept and apply to various situations and tasks in her life. I suggested that she read a book by the psychoanalyst Bruno Bettelheim called *The Good Enough Parent*. In it, he argues that most parents aren't perfect. But most well-intentioned parents are good enough. They do their job well. And there is a difference between doing a job well and doing it perfectly. There is *always* a flaw in what we do. We are not perfect. We are not gods. We are neither all-knowing nor all-powerful. So how can we always do everything perfectly? I have asked more than one parent to read Bettelheim's book. In Jelena's case she was not a parent yet, but she still got the general message and philosophy. She began to apply it to her life, and she became somewhat less demanding of herself.

Whatever you are doing—taking a class, raising a child, washing a car, dressing for a party, or writing a letter—if you expect perfection every time, you are placing yourself under great stress. This search for perfection is also time-consuming, because you will likely either go slowly or repeat work that has already been done. It's not only time-consuming, it's exhausting! (Again, remember that neurotic people often complain of fatigue. The demand for perfection is a contributing factor.) Instead of thinking in terms of a 100 percent job, think in terms of a 95 percent job or a 90 percent job. I have been a teacher for a long time. I give students an A on an examination if they score 95 percent or even 90 percent. Give yourself a mental A for the things you do in this life, even if they don't reach the 100 percent level.

### Coping with Being Overly Responsible

REFLECT ON THIS SAYING:
"LIFE IS TOO SERIOUS TO TAKE IT SERIOUSLY."

As I said before, overly responsible people take life too seriously. An effective psychological antidote to this tendency is to memorize this saying. It may seem to be paradoxical. But let us take the saying's advice and seriously reflect on it for a moment. Life is serious. Of course it is. A lot is at stake. You want to achieve your goals. You want to find some level of self-fulfillment. You want to find meaning in life. These are all legitimate aspirations. Yet if you try too hard, you will defeat your purpose. The intensity of your striving will defeat your purpose. This is the paradox. The saying, in its seeming absurdity, makes an important distinction between life being serious and *taking* it too seriously. Indeed, because life is so serious a matter, its weight must be lightened to some extent by a broader outlook, one that contains an element of self-forgiveness and a reasonable sense of humor.

When you find that you are being responsible to a fault, when you are trying to keep everybody happy but yourself, say consciously and deliberately in your own mind, "Life is too serious to take it seriously."

## Coping with Irrational Thinking

### CHALLENGE THE RATIONALITY OF YOUR OWN THOUGHTS.

Most people take for granted that what they think is rational. We are used to our own thoughts and their patterns. They seem logical and reasonable to us. However, if you stop and reflect on your thoughts you will sometimes find that they are not actually a good fit to reality. They actually conform to your wishes and your fears, to your neurotic tendencies.

Let's return to Rita and Harley. Rita thought, "I'm a failure as a mother." Harley thought, "Nothing ever goes right in my life." Both of them then learned to challenge the rationality of their own thoughts. They developed a habit of saying to themselves after they had a thought, "Is this an example of either-or thinking? Am I employing catastrophic thinking? Am I overgeneralizing and oversimplifying? Am I making a cognitive error?" These questions set up an automatic process of reflection. Both individuals learned that they could modify their thoughts. And, in consequence, they felt better at an emotional level.

Rita saw that she failed her children in some ways. But she was also successful in some ways. She was not a Failure with a capital F. She was just a person who had occasional failures in her efforts to be an effective parent. Who doesn't?

Challenging the rationality of your own thoughts will help you see that life is multidimensional and that it shouldn't be oversimplified.

---

**MASTER STRATEGY 4**

### Affirm that you can learn to cope effectively with neurotic disadvantages.

Recognize fully that you can either neutralize their adverse effects or, in some cases, turn them into long-term advantages. Recall what Nietzsche said: "That which does not destroy me strengthens me." Nietzsche was emphasizing the ability of human beings to think and to derive benefit from experience. In keeping with the general theme of this book, look upon neurotic disadvantages not as afflictions, but as challenges. Use them to grow and to become a more effective person.

---

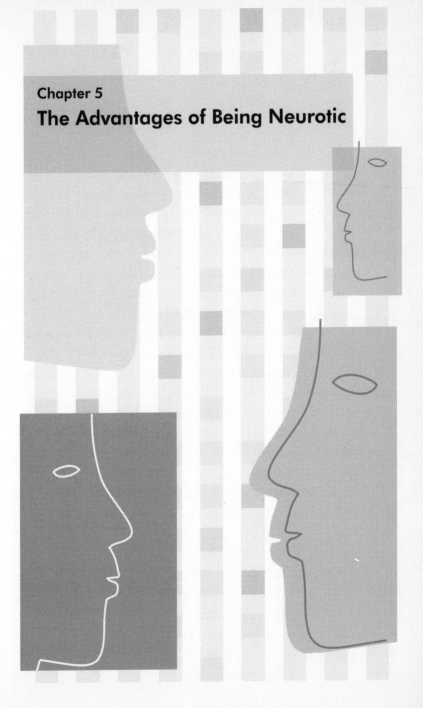

Chapter 5
# The Advantages of Being Neurotic

**Celeste W., a divorced woman** with two children and a job she didn't like, sat in my office and said, "Why was I ever born? I'm so miserable. There are so many things to do in the day I can't stand it. My life is down the tubes. I know I'm whining and complaining, but I can't help it. I'm neurotic and I know it. And that only makes matters worse. If I could only be rid of this neurosis, I would be so much happier. It's like a heavy weight on my shoulders. It just drags me down and adds to my misery. There's nothing good about it."

Like Celeste, many a neurotic person has wished to be free of his or her neurosis. Nonetheless, Celeste was wrong when she said that there's nothing good about her neurosis. In psychotherapy it was possible to help Celeste appreciate some of the advantages of her neurosis and to draw strength from them.

I started Chapter 4 by saying that the disadvantages of being neurotic are transparent. Celeste's remarks show how true this is.

On the other hand, the advantages of being neurotic are opaque. They are, at first, hard to see. Nonetheless, they are there. You want to be aware of these advantages because they will make you recognize that your neuroticism is by no means all bad. As we've discussed, it's a good idea to look on being neurotic as a challenge, not an affliction. This chapter gives sharper focus to this point.

Nonetheless, each advantage we'll discuss does have its downside, a potential psychological backlash. We will need to explore the ways that you can retain the positive features of your neurotic advantages and avoid their potential for emotional self-injury. The second half of this chapter is devoted to retaining the benefit of neurotic advantages.

## Common Neurotic Advantages

Your neurotic personality carries with it a set of traits that have real value; some of them can even significantly improve the quality of your life. In this section, we'll select and identify some of these traits.

### *Morality*

If you are neurotic, you are likely to be more moral than many other people. You are likely to be law-abiding, honest, and generally a highly decent person. Why is this so? To explain this, you first need to understand where your neurosis is coming from. In this regard, Freud's psychoanalytic theory of personality can be very helpful.

As we discussed, Freud said that neurotic anxiety arises from a conflict between the id and the superego. The *id* is the primitive, inborn self. It is the source of wishes, including forbidden ones. The *superego* is the moral self. It is the inner watchdog, the guardian of society's values. Much of your neurotic anxiety arises from the fact that you fear you will actually act in an immoral or irresponsible way, that the forbidden wishes of the id will take over and make you do something that you will eventually regret. If you are highly neurotic, you will probably walk the straight and narrow all of your life. Much of your anxiety is groundless. That's why it's neurotic. If it had a genuine basis, it would be realistic, not neurotic, anxiety.

Be grateful that you have a well-developed superego. It contributes to making you the fine, upstanding person that you almost certainly are. It is Celeste's superego that insists that her children are fed nutritious meals and that she give her employer good value for her paycheck even though her job is far from an ideal one. These actions, although demanding, also have the effect of maintaining Celeste's self-esteem.

The researcher Lawrence Kohlberg discovered that there are three levels of morality:

1. The *preconventional* level is associated with preschool children. They are power oriented. Might makes right. It is right to do something if you can get away with it. For example, it's right to take a dollar bill from Mom's purse if you won't get caught. This level is also associated with the psychopathic personality, a personality that has little or no superego development.

2. The *conventional* level is associated with most adults. They are oriented toward law and order. It is right to do something if it is legal. It is wrong to do something if it's illegal. If asked why one must stop at a red light, they answer, "Because it's the law. And if you break the law, you have to pay a fine."

3. The *postconventional* level is associated with a minority of adults. These adults are oriented toward principles. It is right to do something if the act itself is right. It is wrong to do something if the act itself is

wrong. If asked why one must stop at a red light, they answer, "Because running a red light can result in serious injury, even someone's death."

Where do people with a neurosis fit into this scheme? You guessed it. Most neurotic people operate at the postconventional level. They include a conventional orientation, of course. But they also operate on a higher plane. They are decent not only because they recognize laws must be obeyed, but because they have insight and understanding into the very nature of why we must act in a responsible, decent way toward each other.

Having a higher moral self is one of the advantages of being neurotic.

### Sensitivity

Sensitivity is a personality trait associated with neurosis. Unusually sensitive people live at a high level of awareness. They are acutely conscious of both the outer world of external events and the inner world of thoughts and feelings. The reason that this is a basically desirable trait is that such sensitivity is not only associated with neurosis. It is also associated with those qualities that make human beings unique, that set them a step above the animals. Think of a placid cow standing in a field or the day-to-day life of a crocodile. Although we can't know their consciousness, it seems a good bet that these animals are living in a kind of dull stupor—a kind of low-level consciousness. If this is true, would you trade your sensitivity for their dull existence?

Lenore N. says, "I've seen *West Side Story* more than once. It still makes me cry at the ending." Kenton E. says,

"When I hear the 'Star-Spangled Banner,' I get goose bumps." Chandi H. says, "When I pick roses from my garden and arrange them on my dining room table I sometimes want to 'cry for happy' because they are so beautiful. They make me appreciate the world and life." All three of these people are reflecting the trait of sensitivity. Being highly sensitive gives you a range of thought and experience that widens and deepens your life. Be thankful for this trait.

### Creativity

Creativity and neurosis tend to be associated. Creativity is a desirable trait because it helps you solve problems with original thinking. It also helps you to be inventive, produce works of art, or be more innovative in everyday life. The relationship of creativity and neurosis is the subject of Chapter 8.

### Ambition

Sheila I. says, "I've always had a lot of ambition. From early childhood I've wanted to be a doctor." When Sheila was in high school and college, she earned As in most subjects. Today she is a medical student and is excelling in both her clinical and academic work. She has drive, well-defined goals, and a strong vocation.

Ambitious people often show strong neurotic tendencies. They worry a lot about their competence and their ability to achieve their goals. Their ambition burns brightly and so does the flame of their emotional life.

Psychologists refer to ambition in a formal way as a motivational disposition and personality trait called *need achievement*. People with high need achievement set their goals at a lofty level. They yearn to excel in a vocation or profession, make a lot of money, have an impressive house, raise outstanding children, win awards, and so forth. People with low need achievement sort of drift along. They are content with mediocrity. Grades of C are satisfactory. A regular job that puts food on the table is good enough. People with low achievement don't make excessive demands on their children. They don't expect much more of them than they expect of themselves—which is not much.

### *Responsibility*

Celeste, who appeared at the beginning of this chapter, presents a portrait, for all of her distress, of a responsible person. She cares for her children, pays her bills, and goes to her job on time without fail. She carries her share of the load. This is true of neurotic people. Again, the superego, or the moral self, being highly socialized tells the individual that he or she must carry through on obligations.

Sometimes this can produce intense conflict. *The Jazz Singer* has been made into a movie three times. The first version starred the singer Al Jolson and is often identified as the first talking picture. The Jolson character wants to be a jazz singer, but his father, a cantor in a synagogue, wants his son to carry on the religious tradition. In the end, the son, being responsible, cannot deny his father's deathbed wish that he sing in the synagogue. Before he is able to grant his father's wish, the would-be jazz singer goes through all of the emotional storms and inner conflict that we associated with a neurotic reaction. (As it happens, in the last scene the Jolson character is able to return to his career on the stage, with the approval of his mother and without guilt.)

### *Self-Actualizing Ability*

Abraham Maslow, considered the principal founder of humanistic psychology, introduced the concept of self-actualization into psychology. Self-actualizing people have a strong need to maximize their talents and potentialities, to become the persons nature intended them to be. Maslow saw human needs on a kind of pyramid with physiological needs (i.e., the need for food, water, etc.) at the base. Safety needs, love and belongingness needs, esteem needs, and curiosity needs appeared in ascending order after physiological needs. The highest need of all according to Maslow, and a distinctly human need, is the need for self-actualization.

Not all people exhibit a need for self-actualization. People in survival societies do not have the luxury of asking themselves if they are self-actualizing. Some people just plod along, relatively content to eat, work, and play. Neurotic people do not tend to fall into this category.

Being sensitive and frequently very intelligent, neurotic people are aware of their shortcomings. Consequently, they are often also aware of what they might become, what they might do with their talents and potentialities. They hate to see themselves going to waste. They frequently strive to give shape to their abilities. This is a highly desirable attribute. It is what gives us people who love their work—from chefs to singers, from teachers to writers. In fact, *any* line of work can be self-actualizing if it fits your unique personality.

One of the dividends of being self-actualizing is that you will from time to time have *peak experiences*. Maslow described these as moments of emotional rapture, when you are briefly thrilled by an experience or an accomplishment. It is obvious that a champion winning a gold medal at the

Olympics is likely to have a peak experience. But such experiences can come to anyone in any walk of life. Myron G., a chef, had a peak experience when he baked and served his own recipe for a pizza with a ricotta and eggplant topping.

Priscilla L., who looks on being a mother as her most self-fulfilling role in life, had a peak experience when her daughter took her first steps. Kincaid C. submitted novels to publishers for more than ten years. When his first book was published, and he actually held it in his hands, he had a peak experience.

It is desirable to be self-actualizing. It is desirable to have peak experiences. They are among the advantages of being neurotic.

### A Need for Autonomy

Associated with the need for self-actualization is the need for autonomy. This is the need to take charge of your own life, to give it the direction that *you* want to give it, to sit in the psychological driver's seat. The need for autonomy, the desire to manifest your own will, usually appears first in human beings when they are toddlers. This stage of development is often referred to as the "terrible twos," because toddlers want to do what they want to do without regard for the requests and feelings of others, including their parents.

We don't outgrow our need for autonomy. It stays with us all of our lives. Everyone has a need for autonomy, but it varies in intensity from person to person. Neurotic people tend to have a strong need for autonomy. This can serve as a positive force that energizes the need for achievement and the need for self-actualization.

It is difficult to accomplish much of anything in this life without acting on your need for autonomy. And that is why it is, on the whole, a positive force in life and one more advantage of being neurotic.

## Living with Your Neurotic Advantages

Neurotic advantages *are* advantages. Nonetheless, every advantage contains a potential for either emotional self-injury or self-defeat. Therefore, it is essential that you learn to live with your neurotic advantages in such a way that you can reap their psychological harvest without paying too high a price. This requires learning and insight. But it is definitely doable.

### *Moral Excessiveness*

🔦

**Don't allow yourself to be dominated by moral excessiveness.**

The danger associated with a highly tuned moral sense is that it can lead to moral excessiveness. You can easily become too critical and too judgmental of others. You can also become too critical and judgmental of yourself. Any failures and transgressions can induce severe guilt feelings that might only be mild in other people. And this kind of self-induced guilt can produce dark moods and depression.

The film *Hawaii,* based on the James A. Michener novel, tells the story of an overzealous missionary. A particularly informative scene toward the beginning of the movie shows him on his wedding night. The actor Max von Sydow plays the missionary and Julie Andrews plays his wife. When the von Sydow character has sex with his wife for the first time, he turns his head away and avoids eye contact with her. It is clear that he is disgusted with himself for engaging in anything so base and animalistic as the sex act. Later in the film he continues to be overly moralistic, and he makes a general mess of the lives of the native inhabitants of the islands. His marriage also becomes a ruin. The Andrews character is nurturing and loving, but it is not enough.

Lloyd W., one of my counseling clients, had an adolescent daughter who became pregnant out of wedlock. He called her a pig and a tramp. She eventually married the father of her child. The couple now have a second child, and they have maintained a solid marriage. After a period of alienation, Lloyd and his daughter reconciled. Today Lloyd is proud of her and his grandchildren. He says, "What good did it do to call her names? Moralizing like that was worthless. The deed was done and all the blaming in the world couldn't change it. It was just an act of self-indulgence on my part."

Psychologists often speak of the importance of *unconditional regard* in psychotherapy. This means that it is essential that a therapist avoid being a moral judge. People have to be accepted and treated as human beings in spite of their failures and transgressions. The same is true when relating to members of your family. You may not approve of what they have done. But you still need to accept them as persons.

### Getting Hurt

🎈

**Because you are sensitive, be on guard against getting hurt too easily.**

The phrase *getting hurt* refers, of course, to emotional injury. We say, "I got my feelings hurt." We need to remind ourselves that it is the self who is hurt, not the body.

Consequently, when you feel you are under attack by another person, it is a useful strategy to say to yourself, "Sticks and stones may break my bones, but words can never hurt me." This childhood saying helps you discriminate between an actual injury and an emotional injury that is intensified by your sensitive nature.

Keely C. is a highly trained legal aide who works for a demanding attorney. Keely tries hard to please. Sometimes her boss raises an eyebrow as if to say, "What kind of sloppy work is this?" Other times he may bark, "Mrs. C., this just won't do." Oddly enough, Keely knows that her boss likes her and in general appreciates her work. He has given her several pay raises and a number of compliments. But the isolated criticisms are magnified in her mind. She has come home to her husband in tears more than once. She is learning to say to herself, "I'm making mountains out of molehills. The way Mr. Y acts is Mr. Y's problem, not mine. I can't take his irritating lapses to heart."

If you are a highly sensitive person, you must be careful to not take the occasional negative criticisms and judgments of others too seriously. You have to say to yourself that you are overreacting, that you are magnifying the significance of the behavior of others.

### Workaholism

🔍

**Don't get caught in the trap of excessive ambition and workaholism.**

Yes, it is desirable to be ambitious. However, a neurotic disposition combined with ambition can lead to workaholism. Workaholism is a trait characterized by long work hours and a sense of being driven. It's a good idea to make a distinction between *having drive* and *being driven*. The person who sets a high level of aspiration and works toward realistic goals has drive. The person who works sixty or seventy hours in a business or a profession, is perpetually agitated, and ignores the emotional needs of a spouse and children is driven. Such people seem to have demons chasing them. Many a ship of marriage has been wrecked on the rocky shore of workaholism.

Otto G., a prosperous life insurance salesperson, says, "I used to be a workaholic. It's a lot like being an alcoholic. I was addicted to work. I got all of my gratification and satisfaction out of it. I've been working on breaking the addiction. I've learned, as they say, to stop and smell the roses. I recently took my seven-year-old daughter to see a Disney movie, and I enjoyed it through her eyes. It was a magical afternoon for me. I've learned that my wife still loves me if I don't bring home quite as much money as I used to."

There is nothing wrong with wanting such obvious tokens of achievement as money or even fame. However, you have to ask yourself: If you lost your money or your fame, what would life be like? Would you be devastated? Or would you feel, correctly, that these tokens of achievement are far, far less important than the deeper and richer process of life? Examine your attitude and values. And if you come up short, re-examine them.

### Being Too Responsible

🍏

**Be aware that it is possible to be overly responsible.**

Yes, it is certainly desirable to be responsible. Psychiatrist William Glasser, in his book *Reality Therapy,* went so far as to equate responsibility with mental health and irresponsibility with mental illness. So you should think of your tendency to be responsible as one of your strong points.

Nonetheless, it is possible to be overly responsible. It is easy for a neurotic person to feel miserable if there is even one lapse in the execution of self-defined tasks. Not picking up a waiting child precisely on time, paying a bill a few days late, getting more than a quarter of a tank low on gas, not getting the dishes done one evening, and so forth are all examples of the minor failings that we sometimes just have to let happen. The neurotic person often perceives these kinds of events as major personal failures. Jordon H., a civil engineer, says, "I tend to be responsible to a fault. I've got to do everything on time. The self-pressure is enormous. It's draining my energy. I've been working on backing off a bit. Sure, I want to be responsible. But I don't want to use my desire to be responsible to punish myself."

The drawback of being overly responsible is that it can lead to loss of pleasure in life. This is a condition that is called either *ahedonia* or *anhedonia*. (Both terms mean the same thing, and both are correct.) It has been said that the filmmaker Woody Allen's first choice of a name for one of his movies was *Anhedonia*. Convinced that this was not a good popular title, he changed the name of the movie. You know it as *Annie Hall*. Note that the initials A. H. are contained within the first three letters of anhedonia. The motion picture shows a neurotic person played by Allen who is, at least for a time, unable to extract pleasure from what should be pleasurable experiences. Various traits, including an excessive sense of responsibility, account for his inability to enjoy life.

Challenge your tendency to be overly responsible. Give yourself permission to let a few things go when your personal burden weighs too heavily on you. It will help you enjoy life.

### Learning to Compromise

🛠

**Don't put all of your motivational eggs in the self-actualization basket.**

As already established, it is a good thing to be self-actualizing. However, even this positive motivational need can lead to significant problems. *The Moon and Sixpence*, a novel by W. Somerset Maugham, is based on the life of the painter Paul Gauguin. The novel, as well as the biographies of the painter, make it clear that Gauguin's need to paint, his need to give full expression to his talent, was so dominant in his life that it led to the wreck of his marriage, alienation from his children, a string of unhappy affairs, and finally to his death on a remote island in Tahiti, possibly as a result of leprosy or syphilis. Once a successful stockbroker in Paris, Gauguin died in dire financial circumstances. He did leave the world all his great paintings. But he himself paid a great price for putting all of his motivational eggs in the single basket of self-actualization.

It is important to meet all of your motivational needs—your need for food and water, love, esteem, and so forth. After all, they *are* needs. You will feel deprived and unhappy if you don't. However, self-actualization is also a need. What can you do?

The answer is that it is a good idea to learn to compromise. Put all of your needs on a scale, including self-actualization. I am acquainted with Joan S., a local attorney. Joan specializes in wills and trusts. For her, the income this brings is the equivalent of putting beans on the table. She also has a great singing talent, and she has appeared in local productions as Anna in *The King and I* and as Eliza in *My Fair Lady*. She obtains quite a bit of recognition from her avocation, and this meets her need for self-actualization. People tell her she should be on Broadway or in the movies. However, Joan recognizes that sometimes it is next to impossible to "have it all." She has a husband and children. She does not want to emulate a person like Paul Gauguin who gave up everything for his talent. Joan quotes the psychoanalyst Ernest Jones, Freud's principal biographer: "The art of living is the art of compromise."

### Considering the Opinion of Others

❦

**Recognize that sometimes you need to restrain your need for autonomy.**

In Herman Melville's *Moby Dick*, Captain Ahab gives full rein to his need for autonomy. He runs the ship with an iron hand. Ahab *must* at all costs hunt down the white whale that is responsible for his losing a leg. And the result? The ship is sunk and Ahab dies. The novel serves as a warning for all people who are too headstrong.

The ship of marriage provides a prime example of a set of conditions that require neurotic persons to restrain their need for autonomy. The need for autonomy is at odds with the *need for intimacy,* the need to have the love, understanding, and emotional closeness of another person. This need cannot be met unless you relent a bit on your need for autonomy.

Pia R. says, "I used to provide all of the direction in our marriage. We had to decorate the house my way, we went on vacation where I said we would go, and we socialized only with people whom I selected. I even picked the make and color of the cars we drove. Good old Russ went along with everything. But he withdrew from me. He became alienated, and I became lonely in my marriage. Counseling taught me that I was giving too much priority to my need for autonomy and not enough to my need for intimacy. I'm growing up little by little, and I'm learning to negotiate with Russ. It's helping our marriage enormously."

The need for autonomy is desirable. But you must also learn to use your intelligence to restrain it when restraint is called for.

---

**MASTER STRATEGY 5**

*Learn to live with your neurotic advantages so that you can reap their harvest without paying too high a price.*

This strategy was expressed in the introduction to the second half of this chapter. In Chinese philosophy it is said, "From bad comes good. From good comes bad." This philosophy is applicable in the case of neurotic advantages. Many of the qualities that spring from neurosis are "good." For example, your need for a code of moral conduct helps you lead a fine, upstanding life. Your sensitive nature pays off in a life that has depth and richness. Similar statements were made earlier about your other neurotic advantages. On the other hand, as the material in the chapter has shown, these advantages can, in certain instances, have negative consequences. This is how the good becomes "bad." Take a hint from ancient Chinese philosophy and look for ways to maintain the good in your life without allowing it to turn into the bad of emotional distress and ineffective action.

---

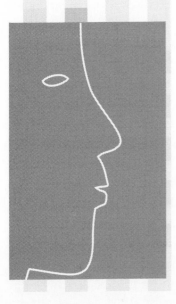

**Chapter 6**

# You May Have a Neurosis, But It Doesn't Have to Have You

**Early in Thomas Hardy's** classical novel *Tess of the d'Urbervilles*, Tess and her younger brother Abraham have a conversation filled with significance. They are alone in a rickety wagon after midnight with Tess at the reins. They are delivering beehives to the nearby city of Casterbridge. Abraham looks up at the stars and wonders about them. The following dialogue takes place:

"Did you say the stars were worlds, Tess?"

"Yes."

"And all like ours?"

"I don't know; but I think so. They sometimes seem to be like the apples on our stubbard-tree. Most of them splendid and sound—a few blighted."

"Which do we live on—a splendid one or a blighted one?"

"A blighted one."

Tess's statement foreshadows the rest of the book. She becomes pregnant out of wedlock. Her husband deserts her when he learns her history. She eventually kills the man who impregnated her when she becomes his mistress. Branded a murderer, she is hanged.

Throughout the book, you are on Tess's side. You are pulling for her. She tries to escape her fate, but she can't. Her efforts are useless. This theme is prevalent in Hardy's major novels such as *The Return of the Native* and *Jude the Obscure*. So it is with the human being who attempts to defeat the winds of a malevolent destiny. Hardy sees the individual human being as a fly caught in a web, a web of circumstance. Try as it may, a fly can't escape. Its struggles make it more trapped.

Contrast Hardy's viewpoint with the one built into the movie *Forrest Gump*. Even though Forrest is moderately mentally handicapped, he has a positive outlook on life. He believes that he can succeed against heavy odds, and he does! He keeps the love of his mother, rescues the emotional life of a good friend, succeeds in business, has a son, and finds authentic love. After I saw *Forrest Gump*, I felt uplifted and inspired.

Which version of life—the Hardy or the Gump, we might say—is the correct one? Do we live in a universe where we must play the role of victim, where circumstance and fate are set against us? Or do we live in a world where our efforts make a difference?

A neurosis is certainly not mental retardation. It is much, much less of a personal problem. But there is a similarity in that either can, if looked upon in a negative way, cause a person to accept a marginal status in life. As you already know, this book takes the position that you don't have to settle for second best just because you have a neurosis.

## Two Viewpoints on Behavior

There are two major viewpoints that can be used to explain and understand human behavior. The first is known as determinism. The second is known as voluntarism.

### Determinism

*Determinism* asserts that we live in a cause-and-effect universe. This viewpoint underlies science and indeed much of psychology as a behavioral science. Determinism says that you are what you are because of genetic tendencies or environmental factors. Every thought you think, every feeling you feel, and every action you take is caused at some level. Thoughts, for example, are caused by the firing of neurons in the brain and by the release of chemical messengers called neurotransmitters.

The determinist says, "If you can understand enough about either biology or how human beings learn, you can explain and predict all behavior."

The level does not have to be biological. It can be psychological. Learning is a psychological process. Human beings acquire conditioned reflexes, bad emotional habits, and even attitudes through experience. The most famous behaviorist of the twentieth century was B. F. Skinner. He believed that the learning process shapes us, modifies our behavior, and dominates our lives. He was convinced that there was no room for human freedom in this system. He asserted that believing we can control and influence our own lives by the application of will and intelligence was just an illusion. This particular viewpoint is summarized in his book *Beyond Freedom and Dignity.*

### Voluntarism

On the other hand, *voluntarism* asserts that you have a free will. Although we do live in a cause-and-effect universe, there are degrees of freedom. There is latitude. There is room for choice. Believers in this viewpoint say that determinists are unable to make their case even within the scientific framework they so admire. Every experiment has something called an *error variance,* meaning sources of causation that can't be assigned to any known factor. In the case of human behavior, this variance can be assigned to free will.

Saint Thomas Aquinas, author of *Summa Theologica,* said that God gave us a free will. However, even an atheist can believe in free will. Jean-Paul Sartre, a leading existential philosopher of the last century, said that we have free will and that it is a basic given of the human condition. And he went on to say that we can use our free will to choose actions that will give our individual lives meaning and purpose—even if the universe itself is meaningless and absurd.

In psychology, Abraham Maslow, father of humanistic psychology, says that we can use our free will to become self-actualizing, to become the persons we were meant to be. William James, one of the principal founders of American psychology, said that after a long period of believing in determinism, he had decided to believe in free will. He was prone to serious bouts of depression. He found that believing in determinism aggravated his depression. When he began to believe in the reality of free will, much of his depression lifted. He said, "My first act of free will was to believe in free will."

### Choosing to Be Free

The free will versus determinism issue has not been resolved to the satisfaction of professional philosophers. There is no consensus in philosophy as a field of study. The aim of this section is not to resolve the debate at a profound philosophical level. The final, objective answer may be beyond us. However, we can say with a high level of confidence that William James was basically right about the impact of a person's belief on his or her mental health. If you believe in determinism, and you believe that it actually applies in your life, it will aggravate your neurosis. If you believe in voluntarism, and you believe that free will applies in your life, it will help you diminish the intensity of neurotic symptoms. You will feel a great lifting of the burden of your neurosis.

Here is an analogy that is a helpful way to think about the relationship of determinism and voluntarism. Determinism is like a hand that you are dealt in a card game. You have no control over the cards you receive. Free will is how you play the cards. This you *can* control. And how you play the cards is all-important in deciding the outcome of the game—in this case, the game of life.

## Learned Helplessness

What can rats teach us about human behavior? Not much, some people say. They can't read books or play musical instruments. They don't fall in love and have an interest in mathematics. Maybe critics of rat research are right. On the other hand, allow me to describe a well-known experimental approach with rats, and you can be the judge of the relevance of rat studies to the human condition. What follows is based on the work of the research psychologist Martin Seligman.

A group of rats designated Group A are subjected to inescapable electric shocks. When a buzzer sounds, they are restrained from jumping to a safe area of a conditioning apparatus. And they must endure an electric shock. A second group of rats designated Group B are subjected to escapable electric shocks. When a buzzer sounds, they have twenty seconds to avoid the shock and escape to a safe area of the apparatus. This occurs a number of times and is the training phase of the experiment.

In the test stage of the experiment, rats from both groups are dropped one at a time into a deep tank of water. Rats from Group A make a few feeble efforts to swim but give up quickly. They will drown if they are not rescued. Rats from Group B will swim and swim and try to stay afloat to the point of exhaustion. The rats have been randomly assigned to the two groups. So the differences in behavior are due to differences in their training experiences, not to inborn individual differences.

Group A rats suffer from a condition called *learned helplessness*. They have learned that they were helpless in the training stage, and they generalize this helplessness to the test stage. Group B rats enjoy a psychological state called *learned optimism*. They have learned that they had a certain amount of control over conditions in the training stage, and they generalize this optimism to the test stage.

The behavior of the Group A rats in the test stage has nothing to do with whether they are actually helpless. If a timer were set and all of the water drained from the tank in five minutes, they could easily survive. But they act as if they are helpless, and, of course, they become so.

Does learned helplessness, first studied in rats, apply to human behavior? A body of research evidence with people, both clinical and experimental, indicates that it does. Eleanor F. has been divorced twice. Her third marriage seems to be heading for trouble. Her words to her therapist during her first visit seem to suggest that she suffers from learned helplessness. "I guess I'm just a loser in marriage—unlucky or something. Nothing seems to go right. Everything I say or do seems to be pointless. My husband has no real feeling for me and I think that nothing I'm going to do is going to keep this marriage from going on the rocks like my other ones. I just don't see what I can do except to accept the inevitable." Eleanor F.

is generalizing her real disappointments in two marriages to her third. The generalization may not fit at all. But learned helplessness is at work.

Geoffrey R. is 80 pounds overweight. He tried diet A as presented in a book by a fitness expert. Geoffrey lost a few pounds, got bored with the diet, and gained the weight back. A few months later he gave diet B a chance. This was a diet associated with workshops presented by a commercial weight-loss organization. Again, he failed. Now he says to his therapist, "I don't think I can ever lose this damn 80 pounds. It's like a curse. It must be my metabolism. It's my genes maybe that causes my sluggish metabolism. You can't do anything about that." Geoffrey, like Eleanor, suffers from learned helplessness.

The fact of the matter is that learned helplessness plays a significant role in human depression. Depression is, of course, one of the psychological states associated with a poorly managed neurosis.

## Seeking Personal Freedom

Here are some ways that you can untie the neurotic cords that bind you, that make you feel possessed by your neuroses.

### Free Will

🔆

#### Affirm the existence of your free will.

Reject psychological determinism. Don't let its logic convince you that you have to live by it. If you seek personal freedom and assert the psychological reality of voluntarism, you can put the concept of free will to work in your life. Believing in free will, as William James indicated, becomes a self-fulfilling prophecy in which personal freedom becomes a psychological reality.

There is nothing far-out or unusual about believing in free will. It is very traditional. Indeed, it is built into our common law. If you sell a piece of real estate, you must acknowledge the grant deed before it can be recorded in the county recorder's office. You sign in the presence of a notary who verifies that you are in fact the person who has signed the deed. But what is the acknowledgment itself? What does it state? It states that you are conveying the title to the property of your own free will, meaning that you are not being blackmailed, threatened, or otherwise unduly influenced. The existence of free will is taken for granted as a real and important concept in our legal system.

Let's return to the thoughts and writings of B. F. Skinner. I identified him earlier as the most famous behaviorist of the twentieth century. He explicitly rejected the concept of free will as a way of explaining human behavior. And he makes a very logical case. Indeed, I am an admirer of Skinner, once attended a lecture he gave in Los Angeles, and have read a number of his books. I always give him a favorable presentation when I explain this approach to learning and the formation of habits to a psychology class. In the next chapter on breaking your bad habits, his ideas—along with the ideas of others and my own thoughts—are put into play.

However, Skinner contradicts himself in three important ways. First, although he asserts that all behavior is caused and determined, he takes a hopeful approach. He sees clearly that his understanding of the causes of behavior can be used to modify behavior. The very term *behavior modification* is inspired and informed by his work. Behavior therapists often use the term *self-modification of behavior*. It is assumed as a foundation of Skinner's thinking that the self can take charge of one's behavior, that maladaptive habits can be modified. This seems to me to be an implicit acceptance of the doctrine of free will without actually saying so.

Second, in Skinner's autobiography, he writes as if he has a free will. He often refers to his thoughts, his memories, his ambitions, his hopes, and his decisions. These usages, all denied in his formal approach to psychology, are taken for granted when he tells you about his own life. Again, free will is implicit in his thinking.

Third, Skinner's life was lived, again, as if he had a free will. He was a bold, ambitious, assertive person who didn't take a backseat to other psychologists. He advanced his ideas, wrote books, became famous, and accomplished much as a scientist. All of this suggests that he had a high level of personal freedom as a human being, that he did not feel constrained by outer circumstances, and that he took his own free will for granted.

Although you can and should take much of his thinking about human behavior and psychology seriously because it is based on solid research, how can you take seriously his philosophical assertion that free will is an illusion? In a nutshell, you can't.

Determinism, although it is useful in scientific research, is a dismal way to look at your own life. It makes you into a high-grade robot, not a human being. Voluntarism, on the other hand, asserts that you are *not* a thing. You are fully alive and conscious, and you can use your life and your consciousness to take charge of your life.

Here is an image I employ in counseling and teaching classes. A Ping-Pong ball is floating down a river. It is helpless.

It must go where the current takes it. It is at the mercy of the vagaries of the river. Now imagine that the ball has a little outboard motor attached. Also assume that the ball is conscious and can think. It can go where it wants to go. If the current is not too strong, the ball can even go against the current. If the current *is* very strong, the ball can adapt and head where it wants to go by traveling at an angle in its desired direction. The ball travels with the current, but it goes in its own way as well. The little ball without a motor and without consciousness is a metaphor for a being without free will, for a being entirely captured by deterministic forces. The Ping-Pong ball with a motor and with consciousness is a metaphor for a being with free will, for a being that has a measure of personal freedom.

### Breaking Free from Past Failures

💡

#### Reject learned helplessness.

It is important to recognize that learned helplessness is just that—*learned.* It is a generalization from past experience. In the past you may have actually been helpless in some situations. But that does not mean you are helpless now. It is important to say to yourself that Situation 1 is not Situation 2. It is also important to say to yourself that the person you were, for example, two years ago is not the person you are today. Perhaps that person was unable to cope with a particular kind of problem. Today's person may very well be able to cope.

You will recall that Eleanor F. believed that her third marriage was heading for the rocks and was certain to take the direction of her first two marriages. Here is an excerpt from Eleanor's journal after she had been in psychotherapy for three months: "I have discovered that I was taking an attitude of defeat toward my present marriage. I was thinking that I've struck out twice. I was anticipating that third strike—the strike that says that I'm out—out of marriage for good. I have learned to tell myself that past events don't make the present happen. I'm a free agent and I'm *not* helpless. Repeat, *I'm not helpless.* Things are better now. I'm making this marriage work. I'm telling myself that to make this marriage work I have to work at the marriage. It's not going to end up on the rocks, not if I have anything to say about it."

Geoffrey R. was 80 pounds overweight. After a number of therapy sessions, Geoffrey said to his therapist, "When I said that I was fat because of my genes or my metabolism, that I felt as if I was suffering from a curse, I was expressing the attitude you have called learned helplessness. By blaming genes and metabolism, I was avoiding taking responsibility for my own behavior. I'm trying a new approach to weight control based on an eating plan I think I can live with. I've lost twenty pounds, and I think I'll reach a normal weight eventually."

Most of the time, you are not helpless. But if you think you are, then you are. The belief that you are helpless makes it a self-fulfilling prophecy. Say to yourself, "I am aware of the tendency to develop learned helplessness. And I will reject this attitude toward living."

## Who's in Control Here?

Place the locus of control of your behavior squarely within yourself.

The research psychologist Julian Rotter introduced the concept of *locus of control* into the field of psychology. This concept can be defined as the place where you perceive the causes of your behavior to be located. If you perceive the cause of a particular behavior as arising from within the self, this is an *internal* locus of control. If you perceive the cause of a particular behavior as arising from outside the self, this is an *external* locus of control.

Take the following informal quiz to get an impression of your own approach to locus of control.

1. It's not what you know, it's whom you know, that gets you ahead in life.

   Agree          Disagree          Can't Say

2. Some people are really lucky. They get all the breaks.

   Agree          Disagree          Can't Say

3. You can't lose weight in a culture that is always pushing food on television, that makes fast foods so readily available, and that emphasizes new recipes for desserts in many magazines.

   Agree          Disagree          Can't Say

4. About the only way to get rich is to inherit a lot of money.

   Agree          Disagree          Can't Say

5. Most famous movie stars got a lot of help from a relative who was already in the business.

   Agree          Disagree          Can't Say

6. Good health and longevity are primarily a matter of your genes. You yourself can't do much about it.

   Agree          Disagree          Can't Say

7. You will find true love if it happens to come your way. It's not something that you can really do much about.

   Agree          Disagree          Can't Say

8. It's impossible to be an effective parent these days. The general culture is too toxic.

Agree          Disagree          Can't Say

9. In order to get ahead in this world, you need to get the breaks. You have to be fortunate enough to be in the right place at the right time.

Agree          Disagree          Can't Say

10. Something always seems to stop you from achieving your goals in life.

Agree          Disagree          Can't Say

As you have probably already figured out, *agree* answers suggest that you perceive an external locus of control, and that you feel you have little control over your behavior and your outcomes in life. *Disagree* answers suggest the perception of internal locus of control. If you agreed with four or fewer items on the quiz, this suggests a strong perception that the locus of control of your behavior is within yourself. On the other hand, if you agreed with five or more items, this suggests a strong perception that the locus of control of your behavior is outside yourself. As I said, the quiz is informal, and you should think of it only as a rough indicator.

From the point of view of psychology, the quiz items are neither true nor false in any objective sense. You make them true or false in terms of your attitude and your actions. If your locus of control is primarily external, you feel like a pawn in the chess game of life. "They" or "the System" or "Luck" or "the Breaks" or "whom you know" or some other factor beyond your control is the invisible chess master. This is the psychological position associated with helplessness. And you have already learned that much of the feeling of helplessness is learned. It is not actual helplessness.

Research has shown that an external locus of control is associated with depression. Henry G. sells life insurance, and he makes a very good living. However, when he started selling insurance, he was a failure. He said to his therapist, "I used to look at the other salesmen and envy their success. I thought they were making more money than I was because they had a better territory, or were better looking, or they were just getting lucky breaks. In the process of therapy I have learned that it was all a matter of perception. I didn't realize that it wasn't what was happening outside that was slowing me down. It was what was happening *inside*. I had to learn to think of myself as the first agent of my own action. When I started doing that, I began to close sales and turned things around."

Deandra M. is a high school biology teacher. She says, "I always wanted to teach, but I married young. With three children and a demanding husband, I had convinced myself that I could never go to college and achieve my academic goals. I thought that with only a high school education it was too late. Can you believe that at the age of twenty-five I was defeated? Little by little I learned that the old saying 'Where there's a will there's a way' is true. I worked out a plan with my husband in which I could be responsible toward him and my children, and I began the long road toward a master's degree on a part-time basis. I went to a community college and then to a state college. I took a half load of classes, many of them at night—later I was able to take some midmorning classes when the children were in school. It took me ten years on a part-time basis, but I achieved my master's degree in biology when I was thirty-five years old. My children and my husband are proud of me, and I have a strong sense that this one life to live is *my* life to live."

It is important that you realize that you have a locus of control, and it is especially important that you learn to reject the idea of an external locus of control. Consciously say to yourself that you choose to take an approach toward life in which you have an internal locus of control. Doing this is one of the ways in which you can cast out one of the psychological pests that aggravates your neurosis.

---

**MASTER STRATEGY 6**

### Look upon your neurosis as something that you possess, not as something that possesses you.

Yes, you have a neurosis. It is a part of you. You can't shake it completely. But you don't have to let it take over and become the be-all of your behavior and existence. The point of view and the strategies in this chapter indicate a way to push the constricting aspects of your neuroticism to the margin of your life. They are there. But they become trivial. They are in the shadows. You will have to work off and on your whole life to keep them there. But it is more than possible.

Reject psychological determinism. Instead, embrace the point of view that asserts you have a free will. Thomas Hardy saw the individual human being as a fly caught in a web, a web of circumstance. You can compare this web of circumstance to your own neurotic disposition. As already noted, try as it may, a real fly can't escape from the web. Its struggles just make it even more trapped. But here is the crucial point. A fly struggles blindly, without intelligence. You, on the other hand, are a human being with intelligence and self-awareness. You have a rational mind and a free will. Your efforts are *not* doomed to failure. By the application of your intelligence you can greatly diminish the adverse aspects of your neurosis.

---

## Chapter 7
# Break Your Bad Habits Without Breaking Yourself

**George Y. is a retired** United States Air Force lieutenant colonel and a decorated fighter pilot. He suffers from multiple neurotic symptoms, including a sleep disturbance and the kind of free-floating anxiety discussed in Chapter 3. In an early psychotherapy session, he said to me, "My bad habits are like my old slippers and my cracked pipe. I know they're worthless and useless, but I hate to give them up." George's bad habits included drinking a six-pack of beer every day, chain smoking, and frequently eating sugar-rich desserts. He was overweight and suffered from type 2 diabetes. So his bad habits were aggravating his physical illness. At the conscious, rational level, George wanted to give up his bad habits. At the emotional, irrational level, he wanted to hold on to them.

George's comments teach us a first lesson about bad habits. *We resist giving them up.* They are often hard to break because they are not only "bad." They are "good" in some way. They pay off for us psychologically and emotionally.

Nonetheless, you *do* want to break your bad habits. In the end, they really *are* useless and worthless.

This chapter will show you some effective ways to break bad habits. These are self-directed psychological strategies that you can employ without upsetting yourself too much—without breaking yourself, as it were.

Bad habits aggravate a neurosis. In the short run, you do get some kind of benefit from them at a psychological and emotional level. However, in the long run, they will aggravate your neurosis and undermine the quality of your life.

## What Are Bad Habits?

What makes habits "bad"? Indeed, what is a habit?

Let's answer the second question first. A *habit* is a learned pattern of behavior, more or less rigid, that takes place in a predictable manner. First, let's emphasize the word *learned*. A habit is acquired through experience. You are not born with habits. (You *are* born with reflexes.) In order for habits, both good and bad, to become entrenched, they must be repeated and reinforced. The word *reinforced* is used in psychology to suggest that the habit is strengthened when it has some sort of payoff for the individual. B. F. Skinner, referred to in Chapter 6, was the one responsible for placing a great emphasis on the importance of reinforcement in both habit acquisition and habit breaking.

Habits have a subconscious element. In other words, we perform them without the attention of our full rational mind. They seem to have a life of their own and, for this reason, unless approached through effective methods, are outside the control of your will and decision-making powers.

Good habits serve your long-term interests. Examples of good habits include brushing your teeth every morning, cleaning up the dishes regularly after dinner, going to sleep at a predictable hour, studying according to a schedule when you are a student, putting gas in the tank whenever you have only a quarter of a tank remaining, and paying your bills on time.

"How dull!" one psychology student remarked after

reviewing a list of habits similar to my list. Well, so be it. The good habits we have don't make us interesting. They simply enhance the quality of our lives.

Bad habits undermine your long-term interests. They are either self-defeating or self-destructive. Examples of bad habits include the abuse of alcohol and other drugs, smoking, overeating, the overuse of salt, compulsive gambling, chronic procrastination, and nail biting.

A self-defeating habit is one that does not serve your long-run interests. Eleni G. says, "I have a problem with gambling. I go to casinos and frequently lose half or more of my paycheck. I have a hard time paying my bills and feeding my kids. I don't think I'll ever have a home paid off and a guaranteed roof over my head in my old age. I've refinanced my house twice." What is the payoff, the reinforcement, for this kind of compulsive gambling? Eleni suffers from an inferiority complex. She believes that she is a plain-looking church mouse without an interesting personality. When she hits a jackpot or comes home with large winnings she feels like a VIP. She gets a big bang, a large psychological boost, out of winning. The hits are Big Bright Moments. The losses just trickle away without too much psychological pain.

One day in a counseling session, Eleni said, "I'm beginning to see that I count the winnings and *dis*count the losses. The wins are what are important to me. The losses I just rationalize away. Somehow they don't sting the way they should." This insight was an important step on Eleni's road to recovery from the bad habit of compulsive gambling.

Eleni's neurosis played a significant role in her gambling behavior. Her low self-esteem and inferiority feelings were temporarily reduced whenever she won. Briefly, she felt good about herself. Nonetheless, her neurosis was, overall, aggravated by her behavior. Unable to pay her bills and meet her obligations, she was driven into an ever-worse self-image.

A self-destructive habit is one that actually hurts your body and is likely to hasten your death. Jack London, author of *The Call of the Wild*, wrote a book called *John Barleycorn* about his experiences with alcohol abuse. In this book he asserts that although he abused alcohol, it was his choice to do so. He said he could quit any time he wanted to. The fact that London died as the age of forty of kidney failure and other physical problems suggests that he was kidding himself.

Mark Twain once said, "It's easy to stop smoking. I've done it many times." Twain's comment shows that he had insight into the hold that a self-destructive habit can have on a person.

## Breaking Bad Habits

In the following sections, I'll provide you with a set of effective self-directed strategies for breaking bad habits. If you will employ these strategies, using your own intelligence and personal innovations, you will find that habits do not necessarily have an absolute grip on you. No matter how long you have had a habit, no matter how helpless you may sometimes feel, there is hope. As one of my clients said, "Like insincere promises, habits were made to be broken."

It is often said that you can't break a bad habit unless you really want to. Some critics of habit-breaking methods claim that they won't work because the victims of the bad habits don't really want to break them. This is a self-defeating, circular attitude, and one that you should avoid. As I've already said, most people with bad habits *do* want to break them.

However, they are ambivalent. They resist breaking their bad habits because there is some sort of emotional payoff to the habit. What they need to do is approach habit breaking in a constructive manner, by searching for ways to increase their desire to break the habit along with ways to diminish their wish to hang on to it.

Although specific examples are used, you can easily generalize the methods described in this section to break any bad habit.

### Willpower

Get rid of the fantasy that there is such a thing as iron willpower.

I have often heard a counseling client express something along the following lines: "I know what I lack. I lack willpower. If I had willpower, I could resist temptation and break my bad habits. But I guess I'm just a weak-willed person." Statements like this have no real content and no substantial meaning. It is almost like saying, "If I had willpower, I would have willpower." The fact of the matter is that the same person who has made the statement may have had sufficient "willpower" to achieve at a high level, run a successful business, work successfully in a profession, and so forth. The problem is that the strength of will that the person does have is not being turned in any effective way toward the breaking of bad habits.

Let's develop a different concept of the will. We can compare the notion of iron willpower to the practice of slamming on the brakes when your car is moving rapidly. It's a bad idea. As a driver, you know that you first need to take your foot off the gas pedal and then apply the brakes softly without too much initial force. If you want to park somewhere, you steer the car toward the side of the road. The car has controls other than the brakes, and you need to manage them with skill, not with brute force.

The same thing goes for the will. You should get rid of the notion of the iron will and replace it with the concept of the skillful will. The *skillful will* is a concept suggesting that you use your will with flexibility and intelligence. In this way you can find real, workable ways to break a bad habit. And you can, little by little, overcome your resistance to breaking the habit.

The habit-breaking methods described in this section are all based on the concept of the skillful will.

### The Payoff

🔦

**Find a way to obtain the habit's payoff in a different way.**

What gives habits their strength? It is primarily in the payoff. B. F. Skinner found that a rat will press a lever for a pellet of food. Once lever-pressing behavior becomes a well-established habit, the food is withheld. At first, the rat persists and keeps pressing the lever. However, little by little, the rat gives up. Eventually it seldom presses the lever. If lever pressing is defined arbitrarily as a "bad" habit, it is clear that the habit loses its strength if it does not achieve its purpose.

When a habit is broken as described, the process is called *extinction*. This is what you are setting out to do— extinguish your bad habits as you would a set of fires. Extinction is an active process, not a passive one. It is not the same as forgetting. The rat in the example hasn't forgotten how to press the lever. It has learned that there is no point in doing so. Extinction is like putting out a small fire with a bucket of water. Forgetting is like letting the fire burn itself out. Unfortunately, bad habits don't just burn themselves out.

But you protest. "A human being is not a rat. We don't acquire habits and extinguish them in the same way they do!" True enough. Rats can't think and break habits by their own efforts. You can. So you have a lot more going for you than a rat in an experimental box.

On the other hand, certain principles of habit acquisition and extinction do operate in similar ways in rats, dogs, pigeons, and human beings. Assume that there is a candy machine where you work. You put a dollar bill in the machine, and pull a lever. Out comes your candy bar. Let's say the machine becomes unreliable. One day you lose a dollar. You pull the lever and no candy falls into the service tray. You stay away from the machine for a few days. But one day when your craving becomes pretty intense, you give the machine another chance. Still no candy. You will now stop putting in your dollar and pulling the lever for good. You have extinguished your habit of obtaining a candy bar at work. Why? Because the payoff you're looking for can't be obtained by your behavior.

If it were possible to completely eliminate the payoff associated with bad habits, they would be easy to break. If overeating, smoking, drinking alcohol, and nail biting didn't provide some kind of pleasure or satisfaction, we would just stop pressing those particular life levers.

And what is the primary payoff associated with almost any bad habit? One answer is, "The habit gives me pleasure." This is an answer of sorts, and there's something to it, of course. But I

think pleasure is associated, and derived from, a deeper satisfaction. I call this satisfaction *relief from tension*. Assuming you
are neurotic, you suffer from a certain level of chronic anxiety.
Your complicating emotional states include depression and
anger. When you perform your bad habit, whatever it may be,
you obtain a certain amount of almost instant relief from tension. This is your reinforcer. It is like the rat's pellet. It is the
payoff for the behavior. And, of course, you experience a certain amount of pleasure. The relief from tension, the reduction
in your anxiety or other adverse emotional state, *is* a pleasure.

Look for alternative ways to reduce tension instead of
eating, smoking, drinking, biting your nails, or performing
whatever other bad habit you may have. There are many beneficial ways to reduce tension. Almost anything that will help
you relax will work to some extent. You can go for a short
ten- or fifteen-minute walk. When you return and sit down,
relaxation is automatic. Here are some other examples:

- Listen to slow, melodious music.
- Take a warm bath.
- Learn to induce the relaxation response through medi-
  tation.
- Reread favorite poems.
- Give an old friend a phone call.
- Go to a favorite nearby spot in a park or on a beach.
- Engage in a craft or a hobby, from knitting to oil
  painting, from building models to playing a musical
  instrument.

As you can see, the ways to induce relaxation are limited
only by your imagination.

One of the principal problems with habits is that they

have become routine channels for the relief of tension. You perform them almost involuntarily because they have become routine and too easy. They have become grooved behaviors. It is possible to pull yourself out of the habit rut and explore new, beneficial ways to obtain the same reinforcement that a bad habit has been giving you in an old, self-defeating way.

### Stimulus Control

🕯

**Identify and take control of the stimulus that triggers the bad habit.**

Every habit, good or bad, has a stimulus that triggers it. (Sometimes there can be more than one stimulus.) The Russian physiologist Ivan Pavlov taught dogs to salivate when they heard a bell ring. (Actually, Pavlov used a tone of a specific frequency. This allowed him to vary the pitch, duration, and loudness of the tone in order to explore certain aspects of the learning phenomena he was studying.) In classical, or Pavlovian, conditioning, the "bell" is called the *conditioned stimulus,* the stimulus that cues the habit.

B. F. Skinner trained rats to press a lever for food. As a part of this process, Skinner had a light in the experimental box. When the light was on, lever pressing paid off. When the light was off, lever pressing brought no reinforcement. Under these conditions, the rats pressed the lever only when the light was on. The light in Skinner's research is called the *discriminative stimulus,* the cue that triggers the habit.

You need to discover what "bells" and "lights" cue your behavior. They can be almost any sign or signal in your personal world. They are relatively apparent and easy to identify once you start looking for them. Mindy A. says, "A bowl of tortilla chips in a Mexican restaurant is for me like Pavlov's bell. If the bowl is there in front of me, I won't stop until I eat the whole bowl." Bailey E. says, "It's the ten o'clock coffee break at work. I go to the snack bar with my friends. They have coffee and doughnuts and so do I, even though I'm overweight and have high blood pressure."

Lyle F. says, "It's coming home from work tired and angry. The minute I come in the front door I head for the bar and mix myself a stiff drink." Laura A. says, "It's getting ready for a date with my boyfriend. When I feel rushed I get tense and then I bite my nails."

If Mindy and the others adopt the position that a stimulus is just there and that it can't be controlled, they will forever be the prisoners of their habits. On the other hand, it is possible to adopt the attitude that to some extent the world "out there," the world external to the self, can be shaped to our own ends. If so, the individual can take control of the stimulus. Here are some options. Mindy can avoid Mexican restaurants. Or, she can instruct the waiter not to bring the bowl of chips. Or, she can count out seven chips, place them on a dish or napkin, and say to herself, "These are my chips. The rest belong to whoever wants them."

Bailey can decide to take a walk at 10:00 instead of going to the snack bar with his friends. Or, he can go to the snack bar with his friends, buy a fresh apple, and eat it slowly while sipping his coffee. Or, he can take his coffee break at a different time. Or, he can skip his coffee break for a while.

Lyle can empty the bar of alcoholic beverages and put them in a far room of the house. Or, he can stop at a coffee shop on the way home and relax for fifteen minutes with a good book. Or, he can remodel his family room and eliminate the home bar. Or, he can decide that the first room he will head to when he comes home is the living room, where he has a piano that he enjoys playing.

Laura can start getting ready earlier so that she won't feel so rushed. The stimulus "it's-five-o'clock-with-an-hour-to-spare" is not the same stimulus as "it's-five-thirty-with-only-a-half-hour-to-spare." Or, she can paint her nails before she dresses instead of after she dresses. The stimulus "well-manicured-nails" is not the same stimulus as "nails-to-be-manicured."

The whole key to stimulus control is to try to modify those aspects of a situation that cue a bad habit. The important point is to recognize that you have options. Say to yourself, "I control the stimulus. It's not the stimulus that controls me."

### Thinking Before You Act

🔋

**Put a conscious thought between a stimulus and its habitual response.**

Often, when we are the prisoners of habits, we forget that we are thinking beings. A habit is a chain reaction with two links in the chain—the stimulus and the response. Conscious thought is not a part of the chain. Perhaps you are familiar with this joke. One friend tells a second friend, "I'm on a seafood diet." The second friend says, "Interesting. How does it work?" The first friend says, "Well, I see food and then I eat food." As absurd as the joke seems, it makes an important point. The person on the see food–eat food diet is not thinking. The stimulus and the response are glued together.

The actor Kirk Douglas wrote an autobiography called *The Ragman's Son*. In it he tells how his father, a Russian immigrant, stopped smoking. As a child riding on his father's wagon, Douglas noted that his father carried a package of cigarettes with him. When he wanted a cigarette, he took it out, looked at it, and said, "Who stronger? You or me? I stronger!" Then he replaced the cigarette in its package. And eventually he stopped smoking. Douglas has said that when he wanted to stop smoking he used the same method, and that it worked for him as it had worked for his father.

Douglas's father was using a method that psychologists call *cognitive behavior modification*. The basic idea is that a thought is itself a kind of behavior. And voluntarily inserting the thought between a stimulus and a response can disturb the usual smooth flow of the habit. Douglas's father was giving voice to his thoughts. And he was thinking that he would control the stimulus, not allow the stimulus to control him.

Almost any constructive thought can be used to break a habit. Lyle can, after he mixes a drink, look at it and think or say, "Do I want to become a self-destructive alcoholic? Do I want to destroy myself with booze? The answer is *no*." Then he can pour the whole drink down the sink.

Pour the drink down the sink? Yes, that's right. This introduces an important aspect of habit breaking. The learning theorist Edwin R. Guthrie said that in order to break a bad habit it is useful to give a new and different response to the stimulus. In the case of Douglas's father, this new response was looking at the cigarette, talking to it, and replacing it in its package. In the case of Lyle, it is pouring the drink down the sink. I used to smoke two packages of cigarettes a day. When I stopped smoking, I carried cigarettes with me and I applied Guthrie's advice. If I wanted a cigarette, I took it out, broke it in half, and threw it into a trashcan. This was a number of years before I read Douglas's book. And it worked for me.

Bernadette G. brought a plaque to a therapy session. She had used actual cigarettes glued to a board to spell in capital letters the word CANCER. This was certainly a new and different response to the stimulus provided by seeing a cigarette.

## Negative Practice

Use negative practice to help you break bad habits.

Some years ago the psychologist Knight Dunlap, in his book *Habits: Their Making and Unmaking,* described a habit-breaking method he called *negative practice.* Negative practice consists of voluntarily performing the behavior, the very behavior you are resisting. Dunlap spoke of it as "practicing the error." He got the idea from studying persistent typing errors. Let's say that a particular typist always types *ht* instead of *th.* Words such as *the, their,* and *other* come out incorrectly as *hte, hteir,* and *ohter.* Dunlap recommended that two or three times a day, the typist consciously and deliberately type the error a number of times—say, twenty. The typist will then discover that when typing rapidly, the tendency to make the error has vanished!

What has happened? A behavior that is subconscious and normally involuntary is brought to a conscious level and subjected to conscious control. This strategy removes the behavior from the stimulus-response behavioral domain where conscious thought plays no role, and places it within the stimulus-thinking-response domain, a domain where there is hope and the possibility of self-control.

Negative practice is particularly useful in the breaking of bad habits that are highly involuntary such as nail biting, hair twisting, and facial tics. Let's return to Laura, who bit her nails. Using negative practice, Laura can stand before a mirror and go through all the motions of biting her nails. She can "nibble" at her nails one at a time. Let's say that she does this for two or three minutes twice a day. This is "sham biting"; she does not actually bite her nails. Later, when she is tense, she will find that much of her habitual tendency to bite her nails has vanished.

Hair twisting, like nail biting, can be done in front of a mirror in negative practice sessions. Also, a person with a facial tic can spend some time in front of a mirror voluntarily reproducing the tic. Willing the muscles to move in a manner similar to the tic tends to bring it under control.

Negative practice has been generalized in therapy to other involuntary habits such as stuttering. Homework exercises for people who stutter include "voluntary stuttering," consciously and deliberately stuttering even when the person has an "attack of fluency" and is temporarily able to speak without stuttering. This is a version of negative practice. An example of such an exercise is as follows: *Stop a stranger and ask, "What time is it?" Be sure you do voluntary stuttering and actually say, "What t-t-time is it?"* Voluntary stuttering has been found to help the individual bring the habit under better conscious control.

You can look for ways to effectively generalize the principle of negative practice in order to break your own bad habits.

### Habit Bending

🌢

**Sometimes you can bend habits rather than break them.**

Imagine that you have a thin sheet of metal. You would like to cut it into two parts, but you don't have the right pair of shears. However, you know that if you bend the sheet back and forth a number of times, a stress crack will appear. If you keep bending it, the metal will eventually break in two.

A similar process can take place with habits. If a habit is too strong, if it seems to have an overriding grip on you, you can "bend" it. Eventually, you may be able to break it. The term *behavior modification* is sometimes used to identify what I am calling "bending the habit."

Phoebe G. had the bad habit of eating eight candy bars a day. Neurotic and a compulsive eater, she believed that she could not give up the habit. I suggested that she modify the habit. I asked her which candy bar, if she gave it up, would be the one that would make her feel the least deprived. She said, "The one I have at two o'clock." She then agreed to eat a stalk of celery at that time instead of a candy bar. She was able to do this. After a period, she was able to give up a second candy bar at a different specific time, again substituting a stalk of celery. She continued in this manner until the day came when she ate no candy bars at all and, instead, ate eight stalks of celery.

Phoebe complained, "I guess I'm still a compulsive eater. I've got to eat the eight stalks of celery. Something's still wrong with me. I shouldn't have to do that."

I answered, "Don't look at it that way. Instead, be grateful that you've been able to modify the habit to the point where it is no problem to you. You've been able to use your will with skill to tame the habit. Maybe that's enough. Don't demand perfection. You have made real progress and this should make you feel good about yourself."

Let's return to George Y., the retired lieutenant colonel. He used to drink a six-pack of beer straight from the cans every day. I suggested that he pour 4 ounces into a glass and add 4 ounces of club soda. The club soda is a cold liquid, and has the fizz of beer. He found that he was able to follow the recommendation. And in consequence George cut his daily alcohol consumption in half.

The general principle of bending a habit can be applied to almost any habit. First, modify the habit if a direct habit-breaking approach doesn't seem to work. Then, you can, if you wish, break the new, weaker habit that has taken the place of the old habit.

---

**MASTER STRATEGY 7**

### Accept that bad habits are acquired and not a part of your basic personality.

James M. Cain, author of *The Postman Always Rings Twice* and *Mildred Pierce,* gave up smoking after many years. He said that he was able to do it based on the premise that "nobody was ever born with a taste for tobacco."

If you look up the word *habit* in a standard dictionary, you will find that one of habit's basic meanings is the specific clothing or garb worn in association with a particular rank, profession, vocation, or religious order. Examples include a riding habit and a monk's habit. What struck me about this definition is that clothing is something that you put on. It is like a second skin. It is not a part of our basic nature. Similarly, a behavioral habit is put on by experience and rein-forcement and is sometimes spoken of as "second nature." But it is *second* nature. Consequently, like clothing, a habit can, so to speak, be taken off.

If you believe that you can modify or break a particular bad habit, you probably can.

---

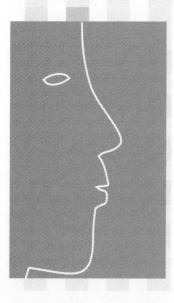

# Chapter 8
# Use Your Neurosis to
## Become More Creative

**If you are neurotic,** it is quite likely that you also tend to be creative. The traits of neuroticism and creativity go together like milk and cookies, bread and butter, and bacon and eggs.

Psychologists have studied highly creative people in a wide range of vocations and life situations, and their research has supported the popular notion that original thinking is often associated with anxiety, depression, and extreme mood swings. Some examples:

- William Faulkner wrote such great novels as *The Sound and the Fury* and *As I Lay Dying*. He was awarded a Nobel Prize in literature. And he had a life-long problem with alcohol abuse.
- The songwriter Irving Berlin wrote such classic songs as "God Bless America" and "White Christmas." He was often moody and had a strong tendency toward self-pity.
- The influential architect Frank Lloyd Wright was the model for Howard Roark, the hero of Ayn Rand's novel *The Fountainhead*. Wright was a compulsive worker and a perfectionist.
- The great comic actor Charlie Chaplin, star, director, and screenwriter of such great films as *City Lights*, *The Great Dictator*, and *Limelight,* was often plagued with

self-doubt and made many impulsive, self-defeating mistakes in his personal life.

- The Spanish painter Salvador Dali was as fantastic in real life as his surrealistic landscapes. He was wildly eccentric in dress and action, and he adopted a superior attitude toward other people.

I won't continue. The list is potentially very long.

The following tendencies are frequently present in creative people:

1. They tend to alternate between taking chances and extreme caution.
2. They have an extreme fondness for the fine arts such as literature, painting, drawing, and music.
3. They like to make things that are in some way different or unique.
4. They seldom accept the ideas of others at face value. They prefer to reflect and do some thinking for themselves.
5. They display the contradictory traits of being both highly organized in some ways and highly disorganized in other ways.
6. They are attracted to unpopular ideas.
7. They are prone to extreme mood swings.

If you can identify with three or four (or more) of these tendencies, and you also tend to live with a core of neurotic anxiety (see Chapter 3), it is quite likely that you are a neurotic-creative personality.

This chapter will show you how you can do the following:

- Draw from your neurosis to fuel and energize your creative tendencies.
- Use your creative tendencies to reduce the intensity of unpleasant emotional states such as anxiety and depression.
- Put your creative tendencies to work to improve the quality of everyday life.

## The Essence of Creativity

Before we explore some ways to employ the union of your neurotic and creative tendencies to improve the quality of your life, let's first try to define the essence of creativity.

Understanding what creativity is, what we mean when we say an act is creative, will help you greatly in making practical applications.

Psychologists have come to a general consensus that the essence of creativity is *divergent thinking*; that is, thinking that leaves the main road of thought and ventures into its unbeaten pathways.

For example, before Orville and Wilbur Wright built the first airplane, many efforts had been made to build a flying machine with wings that flapped. These devices were called "ornithopters." (The prefix *ornitho* refers to birds.) The idea of large person-carrying machines with flapping wings is absurd to us, but it seemed to make sense about a hundred years ago.

The Wright brothers (and other pioneers) recognized that a wing does not have to flap. It can be stationary if the wind over it can be supplied by a source other than flapping. Such a source is a propeller. In order to realize that a wing need not move, the Wright brothers needed to use divergent thinking. They saw wings in a new and different way.

Here is another example of divergent thinking. In a research study on creativity in children, the subjects were given these instructions: "Draw a picture of children playing in a schoolyard."

Most of the children drew, as best they could, what you would normally expect. One child drew a picture of boys and girls playing on swings. A second child drew a picture of a baseball game. However, one child turned in a blank piece of paper. The researchers were briefly baffled. Then one of them noticed there was a caption at the bottom of the sheet. The caption said, "A picture of children playing in a schoolyard in a blizzard." This was judged to be a highly creative response.

Creativity is not the same as intelligence. The core feature of intelligence is *convergent thinking,* that is, thinking that stays on the main road. This kind of thinking tends to be quite rational.

Divergent thinking all by itself does not produce what we think of as creativity. A preschooler banging on a piano displays divergent behavior, but we would not consider such banging creative in any constructive sense. A jazz pianist who produces unexpected innovations is using divergent thinking. However, the divergent is also rational—intelligent—and within the rules of harmony.

When the Wright brothers invented the airplane, an element of divergent thinking was, as already indicated, essential. But they also had to employ intelligence and follow certain principles of design and mechanics in order for the thing actually to fly.

In a nutshell, creativity is a happy blend of divergent and convergent thinking. Although being neurotic tends to spontaneously induce divergent thinking in many of us, it does have to be tempered with an element of reason.

The vision of the highly creative person as a completely eccentric, totally maladjusted individual is wrong. Research has shown that although highly creative people have more neurotic weaknesses than people in general do, they also tend to have more inner resources, more strengths, to offset these weaknesses than most others do.

## Adding Creativity to Your Life

With this background, let's consider how you can combine neurotic and creative tendencies in your life. The aim of such applications is to increase your creativity, improve your personal effectiveness, and enhance the general quality of your life.

### *Works of Art*

💡

**Turn your emotional problems into works of art.**

A work of art may be a story, a novel, a poem, a song, a painting, a sculpture, or something similar. Follow your natural inclinations and talents. You will take pleasure in producing something unique, something that is an expression of your personality. And you will also find that turning your feelings into works of art will give you a greater sense of control over your emotional life. You will discharge the negative energy stored within you in a harmless—indeed, a constructive—way.

Howard S., a veteran of the Vietnam War, suffered from post-traumatic stress syndrome. He was bothered with insomnia, had nightmares about the conflict, and had frequent stomach pains. Seven years after the war ended, he wrote a novel about his experiences. Although he never sold the novel, he found that the act of writing it relieved him of much of his pent-up anger and emotional confusion. His symptoms became much milder.

In my own case, I am an unpublished songwriter. I write both words and music. Songwriting is a hobby that allows me to express my thoughts and feelings, both positive and negative, in a creative, constructive way. When I was feeling particularly depressed one week a few years ago, I wrote a song called "I Like to Be Blue." Here's the lyric:

I like to be blue.
It's easy to see
I seem to enjoy
My misery.

I'm more than content
To sit in my room
Crying all night
Hugging the gloom.

I don't understand
My feelings at all.
I know I should give friends
A telephone call.

But then I might smile.
And that wouldn't do.
'Cause ever since you went away
I like to be blue.

Shortly after completing the song, I called a friend, smiled, and felt a lot better.

Irving Berlin's first wife died unexpectedly when she was quite young. Despondent, Berlin eventually wrote one of his most touching songs, "When I Lost You." Writing the song helped him resolve his grief.

The artist Salvador Dali turned his gloomy, confused view of life into a series of paintings. I am convinced that his creative acts helped him maintain a modicum of emotional stability. In spite of his many eccentricities, he lived a long, productive life.

### Obtaining Recognition

🍂

#### Don't hide your light under a bushel.

It is a natural inclination to want to obtain some recognition when you produce a work of art. You want it to be read by others or you want to display it. Unfortunately, many creative people, being also neurotic, conceal their accomplishments. Neurotic people are often overly inhibited and self-conscious. They sometimes convince themselves that their productions are worthless and that they have no talent. In part, this is because they hate to be judged by others.

Also, there is a false sense of modesty attached to the tendency to conceal one's artistic productions. It is not genteel to advertise oneself, to toot one's own horn. However, as Gene Fowler, author of a biography of the actor John Barrymore, once remarked, "If you don't toot your own horn, it will not be tooteth!"

The poet Emily Dickinson was shy and retiring. She is

considered to be one of our great poets. She was so unsure of herself that only two poems were published in her lifetime. She wrote almost two thousand! Discovered after her death, they set a standard for excellence.

Erica Jong, the author of *Fear of Flying,* also writes poetry. She has described how she compulsively typed and retyped the first poem she submitted to a magazine. (This was before the days of word processors.) She hesitated to submit the poem for publication. When she finally did send it in, she obtained a quick acceptance.

I play and sing my songs for my friends and family. I often ask, "Do you want to hear a new song I wrote?" I'm fairly selective and try not to bore people with more than two or three songs (the new one and a couple of old ones) at a time. People close to me just consider my tendency to give musical performances one of my idiosyncrasies. I encourage you to realize that we all have them, and that it is OK to give them at least some expression.

If you have produced a story or novel, let *someone* read it. Show it to a close friend, join a writer's group, or mail it out for publication. If you have made a painting, hang it up in your home. If and when you have a little more confidence, have it hung in an art gallery. Felix, a forty-four-year-old electrical engineer, started painting landscapes about seven years ago. He recently mustered the courage to ask a gallery to display three of his paintings for sale on consignment. Much to his pleasure and surprise, one of the paintings sold at a fair price within two weeks.

Obtaining recognition for your works of art will help build your self-esteem. Perhaps you are thinking, "If I had self-confidence, I would act in the way that is being suggested. But I don't. I can't put the cart before the horse."

Believe me, putting the cart before the horse is often a very good idea. Research on assertiveness training has clearly demonstrated that if people act as if they have self-confidence, the positive consequences of acting in a positive manner will feed back on their personality and build genuine self-confidence. The behavior becomes a self-fulfilling prophecy. It is possible to act before you actually feel like acting in a particular way. This is based on a very solid theory of emotions called the James-Lange theory, which states that actions induce feelings. In other words, if you act as if you are confident, little by little you will become confident. Put this theory to work in your own life and you won't be disappointed.

### Acting

Explore the possibilities of expression associated with acting.

Acting is a highly creative kind of behavior that is a good means of expression for many neurotic people. You may be thinking, "Become an actor! Me! But I'm shy. I wouldn't be able to stand all those people looking at me!"

Many shy people are attracted to acting because playing a role allows them to express feelings they would not otherwise express. It also allows them to hide behind a mask. Believe it or not, it is "safe" to adopt a false persona, an identity that is not one's own. Self-confidence can build slowly in the psychologically protected environment.

It is well known that people who stutter do so with more severity when they are particularly anxious. It is also well known that people who stutter often do not stutter when they sing or act. The things being said are not being said by the person but by an assumed identity. Consequently, they don't feel as judged as they often do in social situations, and they have some psychological latitude that will help them overcome inferiority feelings. Odd as it sound, acting a part in a play often tends to reduce overall chronic anxiety.

Take a community college acting class in the evening. Or try out for a small part in a local play. If you have talent and want to pursue acting as a career or vocation, that may be an option. However, the point is not to make money or to discover a full-time career track. The point is simply to use your creative tendencies to improve your overall self-confidence and sense of personal power.

### Unlikely Sources for Positive Feelings

🍶

#### Do some creative reading—or watching, or listening.

One surprisingly effective way for dealing with your neurosis is what I call "creative reading." By creative reading I mean reading that is *not* the kind of reading that common sense tells you will help you cope with your neurosis. Common sense says that you should read cheerful things. But creative thinking, being divergent, departs from common sense. Using what is sometimes called "crazy logic," creative reading involves reading something that appears to be filled with doom and gloom.

*The World as Will and Idea*, published in 1819 by the philosopher Arthur Schopenhauer, provides a good example. The writing is dense and often obscure. However, many of his examples are clear and excellent. Schopenhauer believed that it is the *will to be* that brings the universe and life into existence. And, he believed, this will is evil. We would be better off if we had never been born. He continues in this vein for many pages. After a big dose of this nonstop negativity, you begin to feel that it is absurd and overstated. After a while, the cracks and flaw begin to appear. You find yourself disagreeing here and there. Soon, reading this highly pessimistic philosopher has the paradoxical effect of cheering you up, not depressing you! I kid you not.

Here are a couple more selections that will cheer you up. *Wuthering Heights* by Emily Brontë tells at length about the hopeless, unrequited love that Catherine has for Heathcliff. The novel *1984* by George Orwell describes how Winston Smith is completely crushed and emotionally destroyed by a brutal totalitarian state. You think that maybe this is a gag. It's not. In the long run the kind of creative reading I'm talking about is more likely to reduce the intensity of depressive feelings.

You can readily extend the principle of creative reading to *creative viewing* and *creative listening*. I recently saw a movie called *The Good Girl* with Jennifer Aniston. It tells the sad story of Justine, a woman with a going-nowhere job as a clerk married to a going-nowhere housepainter husband who smokes marijuana after a day's work. She becomes pregnant after being charmed by the odd affections of a self-destructive young man who calls himself Holden, inspired by Holden Caulfield, the central character of J. D. Salinger's novel *The Catcher in the Rye*. I felt cheerful for at least forty-eight hours after watching this rather odd movie. Quirky, you say? Of course. I'm neurotic. But so are you.

For creative listening try the soundtrack to *West Side Story*, a musical version of the Romeo and Juliet story. Or select *La Traviata*, an Italian opera based on the story of Camille, a courtesan who finds true love and then dies of tuberculosis.

The existential psychiatrist Viktor Frankl called the phenomenon I'm describing *paradoxical intention.* Are you already convinced that it works? You don't have to be. Experiment and see how this particular creative approach works for you.

### Practical Uses for Creativity

🔑

### Look for creative solutions to everyday problems.

Your neurotic traits can create everyday problems for you. Fortunately, you can fight fire with fire. You can employ your neurotic creativity to solve the same problems induced by your neurosis.

Norman R., one of my counseling clients, related the following:

> When my wife cooks meat sauce for spaghetti on Sundays we have a problem with flies in the kitchen and the adjacent dinette. Don't ask me where the flies come from. It's a mystery. We have intact screens and keep the windows closed. Anyway, six or seven flies usually show up over a period of an hour or so. And my wife asks me to kill them.
>
> It so happens that I hate to swat flies. I'm very squeamish about it. I feel like throwing up when the swatter hits them and—well, you get the idea.
>
> I kept looking for a better way to deal with the problem. Flies are apparently attracted to light, and they usually visit the window in the dinette where I have an unrestricted shot at them. I hit upon the idea of filling a

spray bottle with a solution of detergent and water. I get about ten or twelve inches behind a fly while it is crawling around on the window. Then I give it a few squirts. The soapy solution covers the fly's wings, and all it can do is crawl around. I then pick it up with a ball of tissue and dispose of it.

Liana V., another one of my counseling clients, related the following:

I have a fairly large family and circle of friends. I often entertain as many as ten or twelve people at a sit-down dinner. I had been looking for a new china pattern for years—but so many patterns to choose from! I suffer from a decision-making phobia in general anyway, and I was sure stuck when it came to the plates.

Then I got the novel notion of buying twelve place settings with different patterns. Now they are a conversation piece. We have the same fun talking about the variety and novelty of the designs that people get when they look at patterns in a store.

Both Norman and Liana applied their natural creative tendencies in such a way that they discovered practical solutions to everyday problems. In both cases the problems were induced by their neurotic tendencies. However, not all of your daily problems are associated with your neurosis. You can seek creative solutions to any problem. Creativity is a personal attribute that can be applied to a wide spectrum of human activity ranging from works of art to everyday situations.

## MASTER STRATEGY 8

### Seek ways to convert neurotic energy into creative accomplishments.

Think of an ordinary flashlight. The energy stored in the battery is like your neurotic energy. The blazing bulb is like your creativity. In an actual flashlight there must be a connection between the energy in the battery and the bulb. That is why when we want to use the flashlight we have to move the switch and turn it on. Similarly, you must look for a connection between your neurotic energy and your creative abilities. If you don't actively search for this connection, nothing will happen. However, if you seek your own personal psychological switch or switches, you will find that there will be a steady flow of creativity. This is because your neurotic energy will continue to renew your creative abilities.

Put the ideas in this chapter to work for you. They will help you become more creative. And the expression of your creativity will improve the quality of your life.

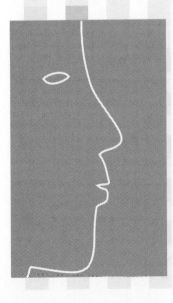

# Chapter 9
# Put Your Fears to Work
## to Improve Your Health

**You worry a lot** about your health.

You know that your worry is irrational and excessive. And yet who is to say that you are thinking in a foolish way? Maybe you actually *do* have some undiagnosed dread disease such as cancer, Parkinson's disease, clogged coronary arteries, the beginning of Alzheimer's disease, or something else. Maybe you just worry and worry and worry without seeking a medical opinion. Or, maybe you go from physician to physician, being unwilling to accept their reassurances. Or maybe you waste your money on quack cures.

Your fears about your health nag at you and you wish you could put them to rest, but it seems that you are the perpetual victim of your imaginative mind.

The condition that you suffer from is called *hypochondriasis,* and it is a part of the neurotic syndrome. It is associated with such other symptoms, identified earlier, as obsessive-compulsive behavior and chronic anxiety. At a formal psychiatric level, hypochondriasis is defined as a tendency for much of one's thinking to revolve around the possibility that one has a serious disease. This is often based on the misperception of minor pains and various more or less normal bodily sensations. The person who suffers from hypochondriasis is called a *hypochondriac.*

The first reassurance that you need if you are a hypochondriac is that you are not crazy. Although your thinking about your health tends to be irrational, it is well on this side of a psychotic disorder, a disorder in which you are out of touch with reality. You don't have a delusion. You are not absolutely convinced that you have a medical problem or a disease. A schizophrenic mental patient might say, with great emotional force, "I have cancer of the brain, and it is rotting away!"

A hypochondriac is likely to say, "Doctor, I have these splitting headaches. Do you think I might have a brain tumor?" There is an element of uncertainty associated with hypochondriasis. You recognize that your thinking is possibly irrational. So your thinking is at once irrational and rational, illogical and logical. In this contradiction there is hope. There is room for you to build on your rational impulses to help you manage your hypochondriacal tendencies.

It is not an all-bad thing to be a hypochondriac. Yes, you suffer because you worry. On the other hand, you can convert your worry into a positive motivational force, a force that will help you explore ways to think and feel better than you do now. And you will find that this positive approach will help you set some of your worries to rest. This chapter will set forth a set of self-directed psychological strategies that will help you put your fears to work to improve your health.

## Why Are You a Hypochondriac?

The normal mind, and yours probably *is* normal, will ask, "Why am I a hypochondriac? Why do I have to suffer this way from nothing—only my imaginings?"

There are no quick, easy answers to these questions.

From a psychoanalytic point of view, it is possible that

you harbor latent self-destructive wishes toward yourself. In classical Freudian theory, such wishes are defined as forbidden. They are rejected by both the realistic ego and the moralistic superego. In order to protect yourself against the forbidden wish, a phobia—an irrational fear—appears. Instead of consciously injuring your health, you worry about it and overprotect it. The Freudian theory is quite likely to strike you as far-fetched. However, it is possible that there is something to it, that it can at least be some sort of factor in hypochondriasis. After all, some people really are suicidal and self-destructive. In a cockeyed kind of way, becoming a hypochondriac is a "healthy" way to fight against such tendencies.

But let's not limit ourselves to looking at one type of cause for hypochondriasis. There are certainly other possibilities, possibilities that are likely to strike you as coming closer to commonsense thinking than does the Freudian theory. It is possible that you were a sickly child, and that you got over your chronic health problem, but you still harbor—due to psychological generalization—a certain amount of excessive fear. Jill Y., a young mother of two children, says, "I had severe asthma until I was about twelve years old. I remember almost choking to death a couple of times. I still suffer from allergies. It seems logical to me that I should be more worried about my health than most people. It also makes me overprotective about my children."

Or perhaps you had a relative who suffered with an illness. Rachel H., a thirty-year-old accountant, says, "My mother died of breast cancer when she was only forty-seven. I'm not only afraid of breast cancer. I'm afraid of other diseases. Whenever I read about an illness, I think that some of my signs and symptoms match it. And I begin to think that

I've got it, too." The death of her mother had the effect of making Rachel hypersensitive to health problems in general. Identifying with her mother, Rachel feels vulnerable.

Rhett W., a fire and casualty insurance agent, does quite a bit of creative writing as an avocation. He writes novels full of melodrama and emotional conflict. He vividly imagines all sorts of dangerous situations. And he has had several literary agents indicate an interest in handling his work. Rhett says, "I'm a classical hypochondriac. You name it and I think I've had it—at least in my imagination. And I think that's the key to my hypochondriasis—my overactive imagination. The way I can vividly imagine scenes in stories and novels, I can vividly imagine myself dying of some dread disease. Last week it was motor neuron disease, the one that they also call Lou Gehrig's disease. In my mind's eye I saw myself as unable to move, the prisoner of a wheelchair, and able to communicate only with difficulty. And it was all because I had the flu and some pulled muscles."

The very fact that we have bodies that can and do become damaged and ill is a contributing factor to hypochondriasis. The anxiety arising from this source is called *existential anxiety,* and it forms a kind of a background anxiety for all anxiety, including the kind of anxiety associated with the fear of illness.

You don't have to pick any one explanation. They all play a potential role in hypochondriasis. And even if you did pick one particular explanation as more or less true and the right one for you, it wouldn't send your hypochondriacal tendencies to the boondocks of your mind. It is a fairly well established principle in counseling and psychotherapy that insight, or self-understanding, is not enough in and of itself to dissolve a significant behavioral or emotional problem.

The odds are that if you are prone to hypochondriasis, you will continue to be bothered by more health concerns than the average person. But you can convert the misery associated with these concerns into something positive, something that will enhance, instead of undermine, the quality of your life. Let's see what you can do.

## Self-Directed Coping Strategies

Let's start by recognizing two general ways to be a hypochondriac. You can be a *nonfunctional* hypochondriac. You can worry yourself sick about your health, seek quack cures, waste your time and energy following false promises, and in general let your health fears greatly undermine the quality of your life. Or you can be a *functional* hypochondriac. As a functional hypochondriac, you can employ your health fears in a constructive manner to improve the quality of both your physical and emotional health. The following sections present a set of self-directed coping strategies that will help you become a functional hypochondriac.

### The Value of Intellectualization

Use ego defense mechanisms to reduce your anxiety about your health.

What is an ego defense mechanism? Within the framework of traditional psychoanalysis, the mind's tendency is to protect the ego, the conscious "I" of the personality. (You'll find more about ego defense mechanisms in Chapter 11, a chapter devoted to them.) One of the defense mechanisms is called *intellectualization.* It is a tendency to control anxiety by seeking information, understanding principles, and acquiring a vocabulary that helps us come to grips with our fears. To some people, intellectualization is a poor defense. Those who see it this way are prone to say to you, "Oh, your problem is that you think too much." Or, "All that reading, reading, reading—where do you think that's going to get you?" Or, "Don't be such an egghead."

For others, intellectualization is an effective defense. Those who see it this way may say or think, "I like to be informed. It gives me a better idea of what I can and can't do." Or, "I find that reading about an illness helps me change a formless mass in my imagination into something defined that I can better handle." Or, "I have learned that when I know the right words to use when I think or talk about a potential medical problem I can somehow handle it better."

Don't be put off by people who are hostile to intellectualization. Looking for knowledge is a constructive tendency. There is nothing wrong with having several books in your personal library that give high-quality, solid information about various illness and drugs. Let's say that you seem to have the signs or symptoms of a particular illness. Your imagination is working overtime. You can look up—as the momentary set of fears may demand—anemia, rheumatoid arthritis, atherosclerosis, Buerger's disease, cirrhosis of the liver, colitis, hepatitis, lupus, Parkinson's disease, Raynaud's disease, ulcer, and many other illnesses. You will become well informed and you will know what you are talking about—and you won't be aggravating your hypochondriasis.

Take a look at what is called the "medical school syndrome." First-year medical students often think they have every new disease that they study. Then they adapt to all of this information, and by the time they graduate from medical school they are desensitized. It takes a lot to ruffle their feathers. They are not prone to overreact to a few signs and symptoms. They know that in science one or two pieces of data seldom form a sufficient basis to jump to a general conclusion. In general, something similar will happen to you if you take the time and trouble to acquire solid information about your body, illnesses, and the effects of drugs.

Intellectualization can be a constructive, useful, self-directed psychological strategy that will help you become a functional hypochondriac.

### Looking Out for Real Health Problems

🔮

**Watch out for the tendency to mentally substitute a sham illness for a real one.**

If you are a hypochondriac, it is quite likely that you will worry excessively about an imaginary illness that you don't have. At the same time you may ignore the signs and symptoms of a real illness. This is in essence a form of denial of reality, a tendency to avoid a real problem for a fantasy one. At an unconscious level, the thinking is that the real problem can hurt you, but the fantasy one can't.

Ursula L., a highly capable escrow officer, was 70 pounds overweight. She suffered from fatigue, the need to urinate frequently, and slow healing from injuries. She has an older sister who has been treated for type 2 diabetes for several years. Ursula imagined that she had colon cancer, glaucoma, and lupus. Now she says, "I see that I was using these imaginary illnesses as a kind of flight from a realistic confrontation with my very real signs and symptoms. I've finally faced reality, and a physician has diagnosed type 2 diabetes. In a way, it's a kind of relief. My ghosts have vanished, and something real has replaced them. My hypochondriasis has diminished in intensity, and my health has improved because I'm doing the right thing for myself."

### Reading the Fine Print

Indulge your compulsive tendencies by reading the fine print on food products.

Here's one behavioral area where it's all right to be compulsive. Go ahead and study all of that information about fats, protein, and carbohydrates. It will pay off. It's the kind of information about food that you need. A boxed cereal may advertise in big, bold letters that it is HIGH PROTEIN! Reading the fine print might inform you that "high protein" means 14 percent protein as compared with ordinary cereal that is 12 percent protein. Now you're not so impressed by the words *high protein*. Just remember that what you need to know is in the fine print, not the large print. The large print is meant to appeal to your foolish child self. The small print is there because it's required by law, and it speaks to your adult self.

If you tend to study the fine print as I do, you will find that this is an excellent example of a case where it pays off to be a hypochondriac. Some will say, "You're just too nit-picking. Do you have to really go after every detail?" However, just say to yourself, "The devil is in the details. All right. So I'm neurotic. I need to know. It helps me feel in control and reduce my anxiety." Note that I said you say this *to yourself*. You don't need to explain or apologize to anybody.

## *Cutting Out Unhealthy Fats and Carbohydrates*

💡

### Use your fears to motivate you to avoid saturated fats and refined carbohydrates.

If you're going to have health fears, you might as well use them to steer yourself in the right direction. Poor eating habits contribute to heart disease, obesity, and diabetes.

Saturated fats are fats that are solids at room temperature. Examples include butter, the fat in and on such meats as bacon and steaks, and lard. Hydrogenated fats are human-made fats in the sense that hydrogen molecules have been added to natural oils. Your body tends to treat them in approximately the same way as it treats saturated fats. Research has shown that eating too many foods with either saturated or hydrogenated fat tends to raise cholesterol levels. This is a link associated with cardiovascular disease. In view of the fact that about 51 percent of us die eventually of strokes or heart attacks, it makes sense to start looking at saturated fats as bogeymen. You might as well be afraid of something that you should really be afraid of.

Refined carbohydrates include ordinary table sugar and white flour. Although such foods as potatoes and rice are not actually refined carbohydrates, your body treats them in much the same way as it treats table sugar and white flour. These foods elevate your blood sugar rapidly. Then you get a backlash called the *hypoglycemic rebound*. Your blood sugar will fall rapidly and you may have symptoms such as lack of energy, a headache, or fatigue. Then you will find relief by eating, for example, a doughnut or a candy bar. And this keeps the vicious circle going. Under these conditions, there is a tendency to overeat. This pattern underlies much obesity and type 2 diabetes. Again, it makes sense to start looking at refined carbohydrates as a danger to be avoided.

Be a hypochondriacal coward. Run away from saturated fats and refined carbohydrates.

### The Effects of Sugar

❦

**Be aware of the harmful effects of sugar on your brain's chemical messengers.**

What I am about to say will play directly into your hypochondriacal fears. Nonetheless, it is accurate information. You can use this information and the fears it may encourage to improve the health of your brain. There is a mental and emotional state informally called the *sugar blues*. As its name implies, the sugar blues is a state of depression either caused or aggravated by the intake of too much ordinary table sugar.

At this point you may protest, "This isn't going to apply to me. I don't eat that much sugar. I don't even put sugar in my coffee. I've learned to drink it black." The key concept here is *hidden* sugar. There is invisible sugar in cake, pie, cookies, candy, ice cream, jellies and jams, ordinary soft drinks, and so forth. Estimates suggest that the average adult consumes about 100 pounds of sugar a year in this form. This is about 2 pounds of sugar a week, and it is way too much sugar in your diet.

Here is the problem. In order to metabolize sugar, the body needs to utilize B-complex vitamins. Eating too much sugar will lower their overall level. These same vitamins play an essential role in the synthesis of the brain's chemical messengers, also known as neurotransmitters. Two of these neurotransmitters in particular have been implicated in depression. They are called *norepinephrine* and *serotonin*. Low levels of these messengers can induce a chemical-based depression. Antidepressant drugs (see Chapter 18) work by boosting the capacity of your brain's neurons to process relevant neurotransmitters.

Sadly, many people are taking antidepressant medication without looking realistically at their dietary habits. It is quite possible that a principal underlying cause of a biochemical depression is an excessive intake of sugar. It makes sense to eat less sugar, to take vitamin supplements, and to eat foods high in B-complex vitamins as a first step in dealing with depression. The taking of antidepressant drugs should be a last resort, not a first one.

You should allow your tendency to worry about your health to motivate you to examine the role that dietary sugar may be playing in undermining your mental and emotional health.

### *Vitamins*

🍋

#### Use, but don't abuse, vitamin supplements.

The old comic strip *Dick Tracy* once featured a character called Vitamin Flintheart. The cartoon showed him popping two or three vitamin pills frequently throughout the day. One well-known movie actor was a modern-day Vitamin Flintheart. He took almost seventy various vitamin supplements every day. He apparently sincerely believed that he could live in robust health indefinitely if he just took enough vitamins. And he told his story boldly and loudly. What happened to him? He got old and died just like everybody else.

No, taking vitamin supplements isn't likely to work a miracle. So don't abuse them. In fact, you should be aware that the excessive intake of certain vitamins that are not water soluble, such as vitamin D and vitamin E, can have toxic effects. Selenium is another example of a substance that can be toxic under certain circumstances. So be on guard.

On the other hand, there is good evidence that taking a high-quality multiple vitamin pill every day can enhance your health. I like to take a gel cap because it is easily absorbed and I am likely to obtain maximum benefit from it. It is not necessary, or even wise, to take more than one pill a day (unless you are taking a vitamin with a recommended dosage of two a day).

You can use your health fears to motivate you to take a single daily supplement. By the same token, use these same health fears to motivate you to avoid taking too many vitamin products.

### Playing for Attention

🔦

### Avoid the "flight into illness."

The "flight into illness" is a behavioral syndrome characterized by acting ill in order to extract sympathy and attention from others. It is also a way to control them. The psychiatrist Eric Berne, author of *Games People Play*, often noted that there is a great difference between an actual condition and the social role associated with it. One can be a sick person in reality. This is not the same thing as displaying one's moods and symptoms and playing the role of Sick Person. The movie *Now Voyager* provided a classical example of someone controlling another person by acting like a Sick Person. The Bette Davis character had a mother who insisted her daughter live with her, care for her, tend to all of her emotional needs, be subservient to her, and live a humdrum life without men because the older woman had a chronic heart condition. The chronic heart condition was as much imaginary as it was real. She finally died of a heart attack, but not until many years had passed and she was quite old.

Hypochondriacs are very prone to play the sick role. The biologist Charles Darwin, author of *The Origin of Species,* was one of history's famous hypochondriacs. For many years he used his chronic digestive problems and intestinal complaints to make himself a center of attention and to exercise dominance over his wife and family. He died at the age of seventy-three. The evidence suggests that he in fact enjoyed basically good health throughout his life. Remember, a hypochondriac is a person with excessive health worries, not excessive health problems.

Don't fall into the trap of playing the social role of Sick Person. It is tempting because it has its payoffs. You can become a VIP—a big fish in the small bowl of your family. You can get a lot of sympathy. You can get out of a lot of work and avoid many responsibilities. But on the whole the flight into illness will undermine your sense of self-esteem. It will intensify any inferiority complexes you may have. You may be able to kid others, but you won't be able to kid yourself. You will recognize at some level that you are a faker. And you will feel worse. Acting as a Sick Person makes you feel like a sick person. You begin to think that way. And you will tend to feel physically worse, as whatever pains you have, real or imaginary, just get worse.

If you are a hypochondriac, don't make your friends and

family suffer along with you. Minimize, don't maximize, the signs and symptoms that induce you to imagine an illness you don't actually have.

### On the Positive Side

🔖

#### Be half glad that you're a hypochondriac.

You ask, "What's there to be glad about? What's there even to be half glad about?" Your questions have a point. If you're a hypochondriac, you've got something to be sad about, all right. You have to endure the burden of living with the anxiety that accompanies your fantasies of an imagined illness. And this is far from pleasant.

However, on the positive side, you should be half glad that you're a hypochondriac because you can use this aspect of your neurosis to motivate you to take better care of yourself. I know what I'm talking about because I have had to cope over the years with a certain level of hypochondriasis. One of the ways I have reduced my fears is to watch my health. I used to weigh—in my early twenties—245 pounds. (I'm 5 foot 10.) I was about 70 pounds overweight. I smoked two packs of cigarettes a day. I never exercised.

Many other people in similar physical condition remain fat or get fatter. They keep smoking. They drink too much. They eat their fill of saturated fats and refined sugars. Many of these people can't imagine themselves ill. Consequently, they are actually surprised when a physician eventually informs them that they have a heart condition or that they suffer from type 2 diabetes. You and I, on the other hand, having overactive imaginations, readily imagine that we are ill. We *anticipate* an illness. And this motivates us to avoid it. That is why I say be half glad you're a hypochondriac. The truth of the matter is that many hypochondriacs lead long, healthy lives.

---

### MASTER STRATEGY 9

## Turn your anxiety about your health into a positive psychological asset.

You will recall the distinction made earlier in the chapter between a nonfunctional hypochondriac and a functional one. If you are a nonfunctional hypochondriac, you allow your health fears to undermine the quality of your life. On the other hand, if you become a functional hypochondriac, you can employ your health fears in a constructive manner. Take advantage of the self-directed psychological strategies presented in this chapter. As you put them to work, you will enjoy two positive outcomes. First, your health fears will diminish in intensity. Second, you will improve your overall health—for real.

---

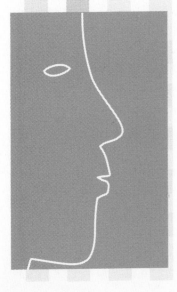

# Chapter 10
# Keep Your Neurosis from Wrecking Your Love Life

**She was bored** with her solid, predictable husband.

She acquired a lover who had a high position and an exciting personality. When her lover became bored with her and broke off the relationship, she fell into a stage of chronic depression. She took poison and died a lingering, painful death.

Who is the "she"? Emma Bovary, the central character in Gustave Flaubert's novel *Madame Bovary.* Written more than 150 years ago, the novel is considered to be one of the world's great works of literature. There is a lesson to be learned from the life of this tragic woman.

"But *Madame Bovary* is fiction," you protest. "It's not about a real person." As it turns out, Flaubert based the novel on an actual case of a woman who lived and died much as his Emma did. However, the psychological reality of the young woman has a second source. Flaubert said of Emma "*C'est moi*," meaning, "I am she." He, like Emma, was unable to establish an enduring love relationship. And although Flaubert did not commit suicide, he wallowed in his emotional misery and became a borderline recluse.

He allowed his neurotic disposition to ruin his love life. The whole psychological process is brilliantly reflected in *Madame Bovary,* generally considered to be his masterpiece.

You don't want to be a latter-day Emma Bovary or Gustave Flaubert. You need love and affection the same as a plant needs water. You, like the character in the novel and her creator, will wither without it. And, being neurotic, you face a real risk that your neurosis will interfere with and wreck your love life. This chapter will provide you with specific things you can do to enhance your search for emotional closeness with another person.

The term *love life* refers at once to both your need for affection and for sexual expression. The love lives of human beings are one of our principal preoccupations. More often than not, movies, novels, and songs are based on this important aspect of human behavior.

It has been estimated that 92 percent of us marry at least once in our lives. Consequently, what follows is written against the background of a traditional marriage. However, I recognize that people in long-term committed relationships have what can realistically be called an "emotional marriage." Also, the basic psychological factors discussed can be readily generalized to either heterosexual or homosexual relationships.

## Human Sexual Response

Becoming familiar with the basic outline of the human sexual response cycle will help you live an effective love life. It is information that throws a little light on what might otherwise be darkness.

The researchers William Masters and Virginia E. Johnson studied human sexual response in a laboratory setting with volunteer subjects. They learned that there are four stages to the response cycle. Stage 1 is called *excitement*. During this stage, the pulse increases and you become aware that a partner is stimulating you.

Stage 2 is called *plateau*. The pulse becomes stable, blood flows to the sexual organs, and there is a general feeling of pleasure. This stage can last from two minutes to twenty (or more) minutes. Stage 3 is called *orgasm*. In females the pubococcygeus (PC) muscle undergoes involuntary contractions. In males, compressor muscles in the penis undergo involuntary contractions and there is an ejaculation of semen. Orgasm is experienced as the peak of sexual pleasure. Stage 4 is called *resolution*. During this stage, you are both unable and unwilling to respond sexually. The pulse decreases, the body relaxes, and there is usually a diffuse sense of well-being.

An important discovery made by Masters and Johnson is a general difference between men and women in the time required before an orgasm is attained. A male engaging in conventional sexual intercourse without restraint will require two to four minutes to reach an orgasm. A female under the same conditions will require ten to twenty minutes to reach an orgasm. However, if a woman masturbates, she can reach an orgasm in about the same time as a male. We will return to this important difference later.

## When Sex Goes Haywire

A sexual relationship can go haywire in several ways. This is a well-recognized phenomenon in clinical psychology and psychiatry. Consequently, a number of sexual dysfunctions have been identified. A *sexual dysfunction* exists when the human sexual response cycle does not take place in its otherwise predictable, normal pattern.

Let's focus on four of the dysfunctions: (1) female sexual

arousal disorder, (2) female orgasmic disorder, (3) premature ejaculation, and (4) male erectile disorder. These four dysfunctions make up the bulk of complaints about distress with sex life. As you might guess, a neurotic disposition plays either a causal or complicating role in these dysfunctions.

- *Female sexual arousal disorder* exists when a woman has a conscious desire for sex but does not find it easy to enter Stage 1, excitement. The older term for this disorder was *frigid.* Many of Freud's patients were so-called frigid wives who did not become aroused by the sexual advances of their husbands.
- *Female orgasmic disorder* exists when a woman is able to get excited and enter Stage 2, plateau. But she has difficulty reaching Stage 3, orgasm. After a prolonged and frustrating time spent in plateau, she subsides unhappily into Stage 4, resolution, without having had the satisfaction of an orgasm. This is the most common sexual complaint of women.
- *Premature ejaculation* exists when a male ejaculates within a time frame that is unsatisfactory to either himself or his partner. Another way to define this dysfunction is to say that in a male-female relationship, it is certainly a premature ejaculation if a male has an orgasm before the female does. Premature ejaculation is the principal sexual complaint of young men.
- *Male erectile disorder* exists when the male cannot obtain an erection that will sustain itself throughout an entire act of sexual intercourse. Often the male will become excited and enter the plateau phase. But then during the plateau phase, the penis will become flaccid. He is frustrated and so is his partner. An older term for this dysfunction was *impotence,*

meaning "lack of power." Male erectile disorder is the principal complaint of middle-aged and older men.

## Why Sex Goes Haywire

There is no one reason that sex goes haywire. There are psychological factors, and there are biological factors. And they often interact, affecting each other in a complex way. To say that all sexual dysfunctions are expressions of a neurosis is an overstatement. However, it is accurate to say that a neurotic disposition plays either a causal or complicating role in these dysfunctions.

### The Psychoanalytic View

Psychoanalysis has had quite a bit to say about psychological factors in the sexual dysfunctions. This viewpoint focuses on emotional conflicts and forbidden wishes. For example, one may have latent hostility toward one's partner. Kelly G. feels dominated and controlled by her husband. She is living with quite a bit of bottled-up anger. Since Kelly doesn't have good feelings toward her spouse, it is difficult for him to elicit the kind of tender feelings that enhance her sexual response. She suffers from orgasmic dysfunction. A psychoanalyst might say, "Angry with her husband, she refuses to give the gift of love. At an unconscious level, although she denies herself the pleasure of an orgasm, she extracts psychological pleasure by holding back from him the satisfaction that he receives when she has an orgasm."

Another problem identified by psychoanalysis is forbidden incest wishes. Freud spoke of the Oedipus complex.

Although it can affect either males or females, it is usually thought of in a male context. (Some authors, when speaking of a female's forbidden incest wishes, speak of the Electra complex; Freud used the term *Oedipus complex* to refer to either sex.) An Oedipus complex exists when an individual has unconscious sexual attraction to the parent of the opposite sex. Note the importance of the word *unconscious*. At a conscious level, the individual is not aware of any sexual attraction. Indeed, due to a defense mechanism called *reaction formation,* a tendency to turn an unconscious motive into its psychological opposite at a conscious level, the person is likely to find the idea of sex with a parent disgusting.

Harry A. was very sexually attracted to his wife when she was young and slim. Now, a few years later she has put on a few extra pounds, is a little older, and is the mother of their two children. Unconsciously, he identifies her with his own mother. Sex with "the mother" must be avoided. With his spouse, Harry suffers from erectile dysfunction. However, he is capable of a normal erection and ejaculation with prostitutes. They represent playmates to him, and are nothing like mothers. This phenomenon, linked to the Oedipus complex, is called the *Madonna-prostitute complex.*

### The Learning Process

Another way to approach sexual dysfunctions is in terms of the learning process. As a child, Vanessa H. was taught that sex is nasty or dirty. This generalization interferes with her perception of sex as appealing. She suffers from female sexual arousal disorder. Let's not be gender biased though; men also suffer from what might be called *male sexual arousal dysfunction* for the same reasons as those that induce female dysfunction.

It's also possible to combine a psychoanalytic and a learning-theory approach. For example, Elizabeth G. was molested several times by a babysitter when she was a preschooler. The whole unpleasant experience has been repressed to an unconscious level. Nonetheless, her early experiences taught her that sex was unpleasant and something to be avoided. Because of this, Elizabeth also suffers from female sexual arousal disorder.

### A Desire for Novelty

The need for novelty can play a complicating role in sexual dysfunction, as a familiar partner may not be as exciting as he or she once was. A person may wish to change partners, in what is sometimes known as the Coolidge effect. It is based on a story, perhaps fictional, associated with former president Calvin Coolidge. A man of few words, he was known as "Silent Cal." One day he and his wife were visiting a large chicken farm. At one point Mrs. Coolidge was alone with the farmer. He said, "See that rooster. He typically has sex ten times a day." Mrs. Coolidge said, "I would appreciate it if you would be so kind as to tell my husband that." A little later the farmer was alone with the president. He said, "Mr. President, see that rooster. He typically has sex ten times a day." Mr. Coolidge replied, "Same chicken every time?"

The need for novelty is, of course, a normal one. We seek variety in experiences. If you eat a hamburger for lunch today, perhaps you want to have a tuna fish sandwich for lunch tomorrow. In the sexual domain though, a need for novelty is often a source of distress and frequently plays a role in cheating behavior.

### More Contributing Factors

A lack of a sense of control can be a factor in a sexual dysfunction. Lorraine V. says, "My husband calls all the shots in our sex life. We have sex when he wants it, not when I want it. If he wants it, I'm supposed to be ready in minutes. If I want it, and he doesn't, he feels free to put me off. And he wonders why I'm not turned on and often fail to have an orgasm."

A lack of intimacy can be a cause in a sexual dysfunction. The term *intimacy,* as being used here, refers to emotional closeness. When partners do not relate to each other in a fully human, nonmanipulative way, it is often difficult to sustain a sense of sexual desire and excitement.

The excessive use of alcohol will complicate a sexual dysfunction. For example, Adrian L. sometimes suffers from erectile dysfunction. When he has had too much too drink, he often begins to think about sex. He approaches his wife, and things start out well enough. Then he loses his erection. Alcohol is a central nervous system depressant and will reduce excitement at a biological level. It has been said that "alcohol increases the desire but takes away the capacity."

Finally, all sexual dysfunctions cannot be explained in terms of psychological factors. Biological factors also play a key role in the human sexual response. If a person is in poor health with an ongoing illness, suffers from chronic fatigue or low hormone levels, or has cardiovascular disease, any of these factors might play a role in sexual difficulties. In the case of cardiovascular disease, many of us have a latent version of this disease. Our arteries are partially blocked, and some day in the future this general condition may lead to an aneurysm in the aorta, a stroke, or a heart attack. In the meanwhile, the partial blockages may interfere with blood supply to either the clitoris or the penis. Inability to remain at Stage 2, plateau, or to reach Stage 3, orgasm, can be associated with general aging and the buildup of plaque in the arteries.

## What You Can Do for Yourself

It may seem that if you have both a neurotic disposition and suffer from a sexual dysfunction, there isn't much you can do for yourself. On the contrary, there is a lot you can do. As we've stressed before, you always have some options and some control. Think of a sexual hang-up as a rock in your shoe. For some reason, you can't get rid of the rock, so you have to either walk in an odd way, or sort of do a half skip, or limp a little in order to compensate. But the important point is that *you can still walk.* Your style is cramped, but you're not completely stopped. This is a healthy way to look at problems associated with your love life—whether they are problems with your basic relationship or with your actual sex life.

The self-directed strategies presented in this section will, as the chapter title promises, show you how to keep your neurosis from wrecking your love life.

### Setting Expectations Too High

🍳

Beware of the idealization-frustration-demoralization syndrome.

Alice R., one of my counseling clients, said, "When I met Terence I thought that he was Prince Charming embodied. I told my friends how good-looking he was and how he knew the words to a lot of popular songs. He swept me off of my feet, and I thought I would dance on a cloud forever. Now, five years later with two kids, he doesn't always look so hot to me. He has been unemployed twice since we've been married. And when he does work he makes only ordinary wages. He takes me for granted and he's much too bossy." Depressed when she spoke, Alice has thought on and off of obtaining a divorce. Also, she had stopped having orgasms with Terence.

Alice's words reflect the basic pattern of the *idealization-frustration-demoralization* (IFD) syndrome. In the beginning of a relationship, people tend to build up unrealistic expectations. Their partner is going to meet all of their needs—both emotional and sexual. People in a new relationship often project highly positive attributes on the other person, attributes the other person does not in fact have. This is the "falling in love with love" stage of a relationship.

If a relationship or a marriage is based on idealization, the next psychological reaction is inevitable. There is bound to be frustration. And this will lead to depression and demoralization.

If you are in the early stages of a relationship, it is good to be aware of the IFD syndrome and to make every effort to avoid idealization. Fall in love, yes. But also, keep your eyes wide open.

If you are in the frustration or demoralization stage of the IFD syndrome, stop blaming the other person for his or her real or imagined faults. You married a person, not Prince Charming or Cinderella. Realize that you may be making next-to-impossible demands. You may be asking your partner, either silently with your expressions and body language or out loud with your words, to be a person he or she never was and never intended to be. Realizing this can help a little to reduce your level of frustration and demoralization. Alice is not yet out of love with Terence. She is working on her relationship from the point of view of the IFD syndrome, and she presently says, "I'm not feeling as frustrated with Terence as I once was. And, yes, I had an orgasm the other night."

Both Gustave Flaubert and his fictional counterpart Emma Bovary suffered from the IFD syndrome. It can wreak havoc with your love life as well as your life in general.

If you have a neurotic disposition, and a strong tendency toward fantasy and imagery, you are highly likely to be susceptible to the IFD syndrome. You need to use your intelligence to work against it.

### Situational Versus Chronic

🌱

#### Recognize the difference between situational sexual dysfunctions and chronic ones.

People often incorrectly think of sexual dysfunctions as chronic states, as something that a person "has." The truth of the matter is that most sexual dysfunctions are situational. A *situational* sexual dysfunction exists in a particular time and place under a given set of circumstances with a specific person. A *chronic* sexual dysfunction tends to be general, an ongoing problem under any set of circumstances with any partner. It really can be useful and encouraging to know that the vast majority of sexual dysfunctions are situational. They are usually transitional problems. When your circumstances, or your attitude toward your partner, or your partner's treatment of you change, the dysfunction often resolves itself.

Taking the psychoanalytic viewpoint, you may immediately assume that the reason for your sexual dysfunction is buried deep in your mind at the unconscious level. But instead of looking for deeply buried psychological motives first, save such explanations for last. If you don't start by considering simpler explanations first, you may wind up thinking that your problem is more serious than it is.

First, let's take the case of the female orgasm. A large percentage of Freud's patients were relatively young women. Identified as "frigid women," they were often depressed, anxious, and nonorgasmic in the early stages of their marriages. Freud treated them from his own point of view on the possible effects of adverse childhood experiences, and he tried to help them achieve insight into their resistance to the pleasures of an erotic life.

But look at the situation another way. Often these young wives were married to men ten to fifteen years older than they were. These men were successful in professions or businesses. Their youthful wives were trophies that they looked on as things that they had earned as much as persons. Also, these men were often used to going to prostitutes who gave them unconditional sexual pleasure without asking for any themselves. (Remember, the setting of early psychoanalysis was early-twentieth-century Vienna.) As a consequence, the men thought they were experienced at lovemaking. Nothing could be further from the truth. Simply put, they did not know how to give a woman pleasure. The crude, but valid, analogy is that of a fine violin placed in the hands of someone who doesn't know how to play it; nothing can possibly emerge but a bunch of irrelevant squeaks. The husbands of Freud's patients bungled the sexual relationship and could not elicit orgasms from their inexperienced wives.

In Freud's defense, he did sometimes try to talk to the husbands. But their general attitude was "Fix her. Something's wrong with her." Freud did his best, but he was working in a male chauvinist atmosphere.

The more contemporary research of Masters and Johnson indicates that probably better than 90 percent of women have orgasmic potential. If they are not having orgasms, it is because of the way they and their partners relate, not a problem that is the women's alone.

Second, let's take the case of premature ejaculation. Psychodynamic interpretations suggest that a person with this problem is suffering from chronic guilt and is denying himself the full pleasure of the sexual experience. Or, alternatively, he has hostility toward his partner and is denying her the full pleasure of the sexual experience. In most cases, these are unnecessarily complex explanations. Remember that premature ejaculation is the number one complaint of young men. Common sense suggests that premature ejaculation is due to a high level of excitement and a strong sex drive. It is a practical problem, of course, but it is seldom due to a complex of unconscious conflicts.

Third, let's take the case of erectile dysfunction. As with premature ejaculation, some psychodynamic interpretations of the problem will cite guilt and hostility are the underlying causes. An Oedipus complex also might be mentioned as a possible factor. Usually, though, the problem is not as psychologically complex as this. Age, getting too used to a partner, excessive frequency, fatigue, and partially clogged penile arteries are likely to be the principal culprits in male erectile dysfunction. If you are a male who is able to perform adequately some, but not all, of the time, then you probably should not label yourself as suffering from a serious dysfunction. Naturally, you will want to explore ways to improve your sexual response, but these should be ways that build on what you've already got going for you, not ones that intensify your sense of dissatisfaction.

The suggestions that follow are all based on a realistic, practical approach to your relationship and sex life. They assume, in order to give you the most personal leverage, that in most cases your dysfunction is situational not chronic. More often than not, this is a correct assumption.

### Respecting Your Partner

💡

**Reject an I-it relationship in favor of an I-thou relationship.**

The theologian Martin Buber made a distinction between two kinds of relationships. In an I-it relationship, you are an "I." You know you have consciousness and can think and feel, but you don't really assign the same status to your partner. He or she is more or less an object you can manipulate or use for your personal satisfaction.

In an I-thou relationship, you are still an "I." And you assign this same status to your partner. He or she becomes a "thou" in your psychological world, meaning that you respect him or her as a human being. The relationship is authentic, sincere, and nonmanipulative. The I-thou relationship is the basis for human intimacy. Without it, there cannot be emotional closeness.

Sexual intimacy is part of general human intimacy. If your sex life is to be satisfactory on a long-term basis, it is essential to reject an I-it relationship in favor of an I-thou relationship. This will give your sexual life a solid foundation.

## Who Goes First?

🔦

### If you are a male, help your female partner attain her orgasm first.

Unfortunately, egocentrism and neuroticism go hand in hand. Consequently, you may focus too much on your own pleasure. Melinda N. told me, "Redmond really enjoys sex with me. He has an orgasm within a few minutes. He doesn't seem to realize that I'm left high and dry. After he ejaculates he says, 'Wasn't that great, honey?' He seems to think that I enjoyed it because he enjoyed it." As it happens, this is exactly what Redmond thinks. Being egocentric, he assumes that his satisfaction somehow transfers over to this partner. A male must realize that this is a totally false and absurd assumption. It is equivalent to the egocentrism of a preschool child who thinks that the universe revolves around him or her.

Remember the basic finding of Masters and Johnson that during sexual intercourse a female generally requires a longer time to reach an orgasm than a male. Consequently, a couple should work together (it's not *all* on the male!) to explore ways to induce the female orgasm before the male one. This can include masturbatory techniques and clitoral stimulation. All the activities that are sometimes called *foreplay* can go into inducing the female orgasm. Once her orgasm is assured, then the male can relax and enjoy his.

The old ideal held forth in early sex education of a "simultaneous orgasm" is out the window. If the female has hers first, the male can emotionally share in it. When the male has his, the satisfied female will vicariously enjoy his. These days, in the case of orgasms, it is definitely "ladies first."

### *Ignoring That Parental Voice*

🌶

## Click off those Parent ego state tape recordings.

According to the psychiatrist Eric Berne, father of transactional analysis and the author of *Games People Play,* you have three ego states or ways you can be conscious and relate to life. These ego states are the Parent, the Adult, and the Child; they are not to be confused with actual parents, adults, and children. When the words are capitalized, they refer to your inner personality.

Yes, these states are similar to Freud's concepts of the id, the ego, and the superego. However, in this situation, Berne's formulation is particularly useful for making a practical application.

Berne says the ego states, particularly the Child and the Parent, make "tape recordings" of past events. Let's say, you resorted to whining or bullying to get your way when you were a child. Today, as an adult, you are frustrated. Your "tape" says to whine or bully to get your way and you do.

If you were actually taught by your parents that sex, or certain aspects of sex, were unnatural, dirty, or otherwise offensive, then your Parent "tape" kicks in when you are involved in sex. It is as if an invisible presence is saying, "Look at you! You're disgusting! Aren't you ashamed of yourself?" This voice, this invisible presence, is an out-of-date attitude held by one or both of your parents. You need to eject this presence from the bedroom.

Think of the taped voice as coming from an actual tape recorder. Whenever you "hear" it, imagine your hand reaching out and turning off the tape. Imagine a clicking sound, followed by a sense of peace and inner silence. You can do this. Remember, you're neurotic and you've got a good imagination. Give it a try. The more you do it, the more effective it will become.

There is a place for the Child ego state in sex. The Child is playful and spontaneous. And there is a place for the Adult ego state in sex. The Adult is responsible. It locks the doors and has sex with the right partner. But there is no place for the Parent ego state in sex. Learn to turn off its tape.

### Of Sadism and Masochism

🔎

**Resist the lure of a sadomasochistic relationship.**

Sebastian G. believes that he has a more intense and pleasurable orgasm if he can insult his partner during intercourse by saying, "You're a tramp, you know. You're a pig. I've never known trash like you. You're no better than a whore." He has strong sadistic tendencies. *Sadism* exists when one person enjoys inflicting either emotional or physical pain on another person. Sexual sadism exists when one person extracts sexual pleasure from the process of inflicting pain. If an individual's sadistic tendencies are chronic and excessive, he or she is said to be a sadist.

Joyce L., Sebastian's partner, says that it increases the intensity of her orgasm when Sebastian puts her down and makes her feel worthless. She has strong masochistic tendencies. *Masochism* exists when one person enjoys receiving either emotional or physical pain from another person. Sexual masochism exists when one person extracts sexual pleasure from the experience of receiving pain. If an individual's masochistic tendencies are chronic and excessive, he or she is said to be a masochist.

Although there are numerous exceptions, the great majority of sadists are males. And the great majority of masochists are females. When a sadist and a masochist find each other and discover they are meeting each other's psychological needs, the relationship is said to be *sadomasochistic*.

The terms *sadism* and *masochism* come from the names of two authors. The first was Donatien Alphonse François, the Marquis de Sade. Writing in the eighteenth century, his literary works describe in great detail the physical abuse of a partner. The second was the nineteenth-century writer Leopold von Sacher-Masoch; his literary works describe in detail the reception of pain and punishment.

One of my clients, Leona M., was caught up in an intense sadomasochistic relationship. She had reached a point where she was unable to experience an orgasm unless her boyfriend had not only insulted her but had actually hurt her. There were times when he cut her and burned her breasts with cigarettes. Still, she was hooked on him and masochism. As I got to know her during the process of psychotherapy, it became clear that Leona had a high need for self-abasement. This need expresses itself as a compelling urge to lower oneself into the depths of degradation.

Leona had been a victim of the sexual abuse of a stepfather. This childhood experience left her feeling, as she put it, "like yesterday's garbage." In her adolescence she had done a number of things that violated her conscience. She felt she was a sinner who had offended God. She felt she deserved no gifts or rewards from life. The orgasm, perceived as a sort of gift of life, was something she wasn't entitled to. She had to atone for her sins and exchange pain and real suffering for the pleasure of an orgasm. In time Leona was able to break free from her negative self-image and give up her masochistic behavior. This, in turn, made it possible to disentangle herself from her sadistic boyfriend.

One of the problems with a sadomasochistic relationship is that what is at first moderate sadism and masochism readily escalates in intensity. This is because, unfortunately, the two processes reinforce each other. When they amplify each other, a sadomasochistic relationship can get out of control. Soon the couple is riding a roller coaster into the depths of a sort of emotional hell.

It is important to realize that in the long run there is nothing to be gained by participating in a sadomasochist relationship. The sadist tends to lose his or her sense of moral responsibility. Often, there is a sense of isolation. One sadist said, "I felt like a kind of outlaw." Another sadist said, "The worst thing was that I felt increasingly lonely." The masochist tends to lose his or her sense of self-value and self-control. One masochist said, "I felt that my life was like an old rag." Another masochist said, "I felt I had no will of my own."

Being neurotic, you may be somewhat prone to have either sadistic or masochistic tendencies. But also, being neurotic, you almost certainly have a high level of intelligence and a good imagination. Use your intelligence to fully appreciate the drawbacks of either sadism or masochism. Then employ your imagination to project in your mind's eye the long-run adverse consequences of a sadomasochistic relationship. This will help you resist its lure.

If you are already deeply enmeshed in either sadistic or masochistic behavior, think of this behavior as a bad habit. It has immediate psychological payoffs, but it has long-term adverse consequences. Turn back to Chapter 7 and apply its habit-breaking strategies to your actions.

### Performance Anxiety

🍄

**Focus on the pleasure of the process, not on your sexual performance.**

Even the great actor Laurence Olivier confessed to occasional bouts of stage fright. Shakespeare said that all the world's a stage and all its people merely players. We spend a lot of time acting, playing social roles. And like any actor, we worry about our performance. In the case of sex, some females may play roles such as Hot Chick, Playmate, Sexpot, Bad Girl, and so forth. Some males may play roles such as Stud, Macho Man, Cool Guy, and Great Lover. All these roles are hard to live up to, and self-imposed expectations may become too demanding.

A distinction is made in personality theory between people who are *high self-monitoring* individuals and those who are *low self-monitoring* individuals. Those who are high self-monitoring are always looking at themselves in a kind of mental mirror. They worry about how they look, what they say, and what they do. They are concerned about the impression they are making on others. Those who are low self-monitoring are more autonomous. They do what they want to do and feel what they want to feel without excessive preoccupation about the opinions of others. As you have probably already guessed, neurotic people tend to be high self-monitoring individuals.

Combine the twin tendencies to play a social role and to be a high self-monitoring individual, and you have an undesirable combination. It results in the same kind of stage fright experienced by actual actors. In the sexual domain, this translates into something called *performance anxiety*. The individual asks himself or herself, "How am I going over? Will I be able to maintain an erection this time? Will I have an orgasm this time?" These self-reflective questions intensify anxiety and interfere both with sexual pleasure and with the very thing they address: sexual performance. Too much attention to performance will actually undercut the performance and disturb the flow of the sexual process.

Direct your attention away from the performance itself. Don't focus on outcomes. Stop asking yourself questions that induce anxiety. Recognize that you are a high self-monitoring individual, and use this recognition to modify excessive self-monitoring.

---

### MASTER STRATEGY 10

### Work toward emotional closeness with your partner.

A poor human relationship results in a poor sexual relationship. If, on the other hand, the channels of communication are open between you and the person you love, then your neurotic disposition is just a minor nuisance, not a major impediment to your happiness and sexual satisfaction. Avoid the trap of the IFD syndrome. Don't expect too much of your partner. And, for that matter, don't expect too much of yourself. You are both human beings with flaws. Consequently, make realistic allowances for imperfections. Think in terms of an I-thou relationship, not an I-it relationship. Don't allow neurotic egocentrism to induce you to place your own needs and pleasure above the needs and pleasure of your partner. Seek love and affection. Then sexual satisfaction is likely to follow.

---

## Chapter 11
# Who's Kidding Whom?

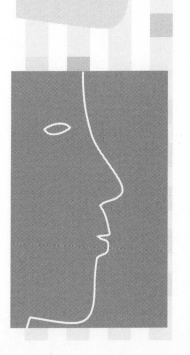

**Human beings are** masters of self-deception.

Given your neurotic disposition, it is likely that you are a Grand Master of self-deception.

The chapter title asks the question, "Who's kidding whom?" The answer is that it is quite likely that you spend a lot of time kidding *yourself.* And if there is one person in this world you *don't* want to kid, it is you. Being self-deceptive will irritate your neurosis and contribute to any feelings of personal misery you may have.

## Protecting Our Ego

The principal way we kid ourselves is by employing ego defense mechanisms. These are psychological devices that steer us away from reality. Consequently, using them makes it very difficult for us to cope effectively with our problems.

Freud is often cited as the first thinker to clearly identify and specify the concept of ego defense. His daughter Anna Freud, also a psychoanalyst, did much to elaborate and identify various ego defense mechanisms.

An *ego defense mechanism* is an involuntary tendency to put up a psychological barrier, a kind of shield, protecting your ego from events thrown at you by the real world. The aim is to protect your ego from the "slings and arrows of outrageous fortune." As I said before, your ego is the conscious "I" of your personality. It is the part of your personality that orients you toward reality and helps you function and survive in this sometimes hostile—and yes, sometimes friendly—world.

Ego defense mechanisms appear primarily as a response to perceived danger or hostility. If everything in life were clear sailing and fair skies, there would be no need for these mechanisms. Think of a modern aircraft carrier. It is sailing in hostile waters. It has an automatic early-warning system. If the system is on alert, and if an enemy aircraft enters its protected zone, a missile will be sent up without consulting the captain.

Your ego is like the aircraft carrier. And your ego defense mechanisms are like the early-warning system. Note that the system is *automatic,* and, as included in the definition, also *involuntary.* Often when you use an ego defense mechanism you don't even know that you are doing so. The use of the mechanism has become a kind of mental reflex, a psychological habit. One of the principal aims of this chapter is to help you catch yourself in the act and to avoid using an ego defense mechanism when it is not in your best interest.

Also, note that an early-warning system can sometimes respond to a false positive; that is, information that turns out to not be dangerous after all. Perhaps the enemy "missile" is in fact a friendly passenger plane. Similarly, Jessica's friend Deborah remarks, "I just love your new dress." A paranoid projection on Jessica's part might be "I know what she means by that remark. She's jealous as usual." It is possible that Jessica perceives Deborah's remark as a false positive. Perhaps Deborah really likes Jessica's dress and is paying her a sincere compliment.

## Defense Mechanisms: Advantages and Disadvantages

On the whole, ego defense mechanisms are undesirable. They insulate you from reality and aggravate your neurosis. They keep you from coping in a realistic way with your problems.

On the other hand, they are certainly not all bad. They do protect your ego, just as they are supposed to do. And at times when your emotional life is overly rough, these mechanisms can help keep you on an even keel. If your ego is completely unprotected, if any criticism or unhappy event can "crush it," you'll collapse and be unable to function. This happens to people who have a psychotic episode, who lose touch with reality. Psychiatrists sometimes say, "They have lost ego integrity." So, obviously, you want to keep your ego intact.

But, as with many things, there is a difference between use and abuse. If you use an ego defense mechanism only when appropriate, this would be effective use. But if you have gotten, so to speak, psychologically addicted to these mechanisms, then you'll employ an ego defense at the drop of a hat. Under these circumstances, you are abusing the defense system.

In some cases a defense mechanism can be stood on its head. You can turn it upside down and make it work as a positive force in your life. You can turn the weakness of a tendency to abuse defense mechanisms into a psychological strength.

## Coping with Defense Mechanisms

This section will help you cope with your tendency to use defense mechanisms. It will identify the principal defense mechanisms, how they work, and how to avoid their adverse effects on your personality. The self-directed psychological strategies that follow will show you how (1) to avoid the abuse of defense mechanisms and (2) to draw a positive benefit from them.

### Denial of Reality

🔦

**Look for ways to face, not deny, reality.**

The most primitive defense mechanism of all is *denial of reality*. The individual simply says, "It isn't so," or "It can't be so" in the face of irrefutable evidence. Three-year-old Martha has opened all of her presents on Christmas morning. She asks, "Where's my pony?" Her parents patiently explain that there will be no pony. They never promised her one. Martha says, "My pony will come today. Santa Claus will bring it."

I knew a man who would keep driving his car, refusing to stop for gas, even when the gas gauge read "Empty." When I pointed this out to him, he would say, "Oh, we can easily go five or ten miles more." He often found himself stranded, hiking for a gallon of gas.

These examples are fairly mild and perhaps even slightly amusing. But denial of reality can have many serious consequences. Madison was forty-five when his physician told him that an x-ray showed a spot on one of his lungs. The physician suspected lung cancer. Madison's first reaction was, "It can't be true." He told the physician, "How do I know this isn't a mistake? How do I know these aren't somebody else's x-rays?" The physician shrugged and said, "Go to another physician. Start all over. Get a second opinion. If a second person who doesn't even know me finds the same thing, you can be pretty sure that the report is right and that the report refers to you."

When Madison went home, he told his wife, "That guy is crazy. I feel fine." His wife encouraged him to take the physician's report seriously or get another opinion. Madison did neither. When about a year later he began to have severe symptoms and spit up blood, it was too late for effective treatment.

You should tell yourself that denial of reality is a primitive defense mechanism. Learn to recognize any tendency you may have in this direction. In order to cope with this world effectively, you have to deal with its hard facts, unpleasant or not.

### Repression

Seek to uncover your repressed mental and emotional information.

*Repression* is the denial of inner reality. When the ego uses repression, it shoves down mental and emotional information to an unconscious level. It is this activity that creates the unconscious domain, often referred to as "the unconscious mind." This psychological territory is of particular interest to psychoanalysis. Freud saw himself as an explorer, as a sort of conquistador for humanity. And the new world he was opening up for investigation was the unconscious mind.

Without repression, the unconscious level of the personality would not exist. Freud once said, "The mind is an iceberg." Like an iceberg, the conscious tip of your mind, exposed to the easy scrutiny of the self, is just a small part of your whole personality.

And just what is repressed? What mental and emotional information is sent to the unconscious domain? It is information that is threatening to the ego, information that makes us feel inadequate, guilty, or distressed. In practice, Freud identified three primary categories: (1) early painful childhood memories, (2) forbidden sexual wishes, and (3) forbidden aggressive wishes.

The ideas, perceptions, and motives attached to these three categories are banished to the unconscious just as political dissidents and criminals in some countries are banished to a dungeon. The unconscious is the dungeon of the mind. However, the "prisoners" are not absolute prisoners. They make noise. They shout and fuss and let the conscious mind know that they still exist. And, according to Freud, this is a process that aggravates your neurosis.

How do you handle your psychological prisoners? You can whip them down, reject them, and hope that they'll shut up. But they probably won't. Or you can make some sort of effort to rehabilitate them. You can get acquainted with them and look for ways to understand them in the light of your rational, conscious mind.

Freud takes the second pathway. He suggests that you make contact with your repressed ideas, and that this contact will help you pacify them. In a nutshell, Freud, like Socrates more than 2,000 years before, advises, "Know thyself."

But how? Short of going into an actual psychoanalysis with a therapist, there is much that you can do for yourself. In practice, this means keeping a written journal of your associations, dreams, and verbal slips. Keep in mind that this journal is for your eyes only. Some people keep their journal, or at least key portions of it, in a personal code. Samuel Pepys, in seventeenth-century England, kept what is known today as the *Diary of Samuel Pepys*. The entire diary was kept in code. Your associations should be what Freud referred to as *free associations*. These are random thoughts that suggest themselves to each other without benefit of logic or a plan. In other words, you just write down anything that comes to mind more or less without rhyme or reason. This is the basic instruction of psychoanalytic therapy. The patient reclines on the couch and says anything that comes to mind.

In your case, instead of talking, you are writing. After you have written several paragraphs, stop. Now look at what you have written in the light of reason. What does it mean? What repressed motives does it suggest? What would your not-so-nice self like to be doing that your better self is keeping it from doing? How can you reconcile conflicting demands of your personality? The answers you give yourself to these questions are your *interpretations,* the meanings you assign to the information that has been delivered to you from an unconscious level. And this is what is meant in psychoanalysis by *insight.* It is the understanding, at a rational level, of what is chaotic and meaningless at an unconscious level. Insight is generally regarded as something that will make you feel better. It is like a balm on a wound. When you understand yourself better, you tend to feel better about yourself.

Thorpe O. is a forty-eight-year-old civil engineer. He works for his father, is his only employee, and his seventy-year-old father shows no signs of retiring. Here is one of the interpretations in Thorpe's journal: "My random writings for the last two weeks have brought me back several memories that focus on the way my father dominated me as a child and a teenager. He has always been bossy and excessively controlling and he still is. I'm filled with resentment toward him and still I keep working for him. Why? Because somehow he's made me feel that I can't make it on my own, that I need him. I'm not sure it's true. But I do know this much. If I keep working for him and with him at this age it's my choice. And the hostility I feel toward him is my problem, not his. I'm either going to make my peace with him as a coworker or I'm going to strike out on my own. I'm not going to be sullen and undermine our work together. There's no point in it. It's just a sort of self-indulgence on my part."

Karen D. is a thirty-three-year-old woman with two children and a husband named Sawyer. Here is one of the interpretations in her journal: "So that's it! Now I know! I've got a secret crush on my brother-in-law. OK, I admit it. I've got erotic feelings for him. Yes, dammit, I could go to bed with him if I let myself. But this is just idle wishing. My rational mind and my moral side tell me I never will act like a fool. I'm just not that stupid or impulsive. But now I see why I act so badly toward him. It's a way of keeping him at a distance. It's a way of protecting myself. I have to stop acting so badly. It's not my brother-in-law's fault. He doesn't flirt with me. I have to recognize that I need to cope realistically with my own erotic feelings."

### Rationalization

🌶

**Be on the alert for self-defeating rationalizations.**

Laverne F. is on a diet. She has promised herself that she will stick to the diet and not cheat until she loses 10 pounds. She finds herself in a shopping center. It's three in the afternoon and she's hungry. She passes a doughnut stand. She thinks, "I better get a doughnut and a cup of coffee. I'm beginning to feel faint. I think I have a low blood sugar problem, and I better do something to keep my blood sugar up." So she gets a doughnut and a cup of coffee. The coffee is black, of course. She doesn't ever add sugar to her coffee. For her, that's a real no-no.

A self-defeating rationalization is an explanation that we offer to the self for our mistakes, our errors, and our transgressions. The term *rationalization* is used to suggest that the explanation has a rational-sounding quality, although it is not in fact rational. It is the opposite of rational, and is, in fact, irrational.

Is Laverne using a rationalization? She certainly is. She is informed enough to know that a doughnut will, yes, cause her blood sugar to rise. But, filled with sugar itself, the doughnut will make blood sugar rise too rapidly. Then there will be a severe reaction called the *hypoglycemic rebound*. What's more, coffee stimulates the pancreas to secrete insulin. And this will only aggravate the rebound effect. It is likely that Laverne will be shaky and hungrier than ever at four or five in the afternoon. Laverne is familiar with these facts, but she is denying reality. Combining the two defense mechanisms of denial of reality and rationalization, she falls into the trap of self-defeating behavior. The fact of the matter is that her forbidden wish is "I want a doughnut." And the rationalization gives her the means to gratify her wish.

Here are some other examples of self-defeating rationalizations. "I got a bad grade on the test because the teacher asked questions that were too hard." "I was given a speeding ticket because the officer was sneaky. He was hiding behind some trees." "I can't help it that I drink too much. I'm depressed and nothing but alcohol makes me feel better."

"I was betting a good roulette system, but Lady Luck turned against me."

On the other hand, one kind of rationalization does in fact have a positive effect. It is the sweet lemons kind of rationalization. The time to use this defense mechanism is when life hands you a bad deal. You sustain an injury or a financial loss, or something else goes wrong. You've got to live with the situation. Genevieve F. was a sought-after fashion model. She broke a leg in a skiing accident, and subsequently she walked with a limp. No amount of therapy would remove the limp. She was unable to resume her modeling career. She took up designing and in time earned wide recognition. She eventually said, "Breaking my leg and learning to live with my limp was not a bad thing, but a good thing. It transformed me from a superficial person into a person with a certain amount of depth and substance. It made me search for my creative self."

Recall that the German philosopher Friedrich Nietzsche said, "That which does not destroy me strengthens me." This is essentially a version of the sweet lemons kind of rationalization. (There is more about this way of thinking in Chapter 19.)

### *Projection*

**Realize that the world you live in is to a large extent a projection of your unconscious mind.**

There is a somewhat feeble joke that has been making the rounds of clinical psychology for a number of years. An adolescent male is shown the Rorschach cards. These are ambiguous inkblots. The psychologist gives the following instructions: "Look at these cards and tell me what you see." There are ten cards and they can be turned in various ways. In every instance the youth gives a response having to do with sex. After the subject has given all of his responses, the psychologist asks, "Now, can you tell me why you saw some- thing sexual in every card?" The teenager answers, "Gee, I don't know, Doctor. You're the one showing me the dirty pictures."

As absurd as the joke is, it gets the idea across. The "dirty pictures" are the subject's projections. A *projection* is a per- ception of the external world controlled by unconscious motives. The external world is the world "out there" in con- trast to the self, the world "in here." The Rorschach test is based on the theory of projection. The individual's responses are dominated by unconscious motives because the patterns on the card are in and of themselves nothing at all. However, to some extent, the entire external world is as ambiguous as the Rorschach cards.

George Orwell's novel *1984* begins with these words: "It was a bright cold day in April, and the clocks were striking thirteen. Winston Smith, his chin nuzzled into his breast in an effort to escape the vile wind, slipped quickly through the glass door of Victory Mansions, though not quickly enough to prevent a swirl of gritty dust from entering along with him." Winston perceives the wind as vile because he himself is in a vile mood. He lives in a totalitarian state and is miserable. The vileness of the wind is not an objective fact. It is his percep- tion of the wind, his projection. To an eight-year-old child with a kite, the wind might not be vile at all. On the contrary, the child might perceive it as a friendly wind that will help with the adventure of flying the kite.

Given your neurotic disposition, you are likely to have an unfortunate tendency to project your emotional problems onto the external world. You will recall from the opening pages of this chapter that Jessica's friend Deborah remarked, "I just love your new dress." A paranoid projection on Jessica's part was "I know what she means by that remark. She's jealous as usual." It is Jessica's low self-esteem, her general feeling of inadequacy that controls the projection.

Be alert to your tendency to make projections that distort your personal world in negative ways.

### Fantasy

### Use fantasy in constructive, not passive, ways.

One of the great attributes of the human mind is the capacity for fantasy. As indicated in Chapter 8, being neurotic you are likely to have a vivid imagination. As an ego defense mechanism, fantasy is employed when the ego seems to stand helpless in the face of reality. The classical example of fantasy employed in this way is presented in the James Thurber story, "The Secret Life of Walter Mitty." Walter is a henpecked husband. His wife bosses him around, takes him for granted, and in general treats him like a worm. Walter takes flight into a realm of fantasy. He sees himself as a brave sea captain, as a military commander, and so forth. In his fantasy world, he is competent and filled with quiet courage. Obviously, Walter uses fantasy to protect his battered ego, to keep it from total collapse.

Neurotic people often employ fantasy in the Walter Mitty mode. Your boss criticizes you unfairly and you fantasize hitting him or her on the nose. Your teacher gives you an F on a test and you fantasize putting a big scratch on his or her new car. You get a big, unexpected tax bill from Uncle Sam, and you fantasize running off to South America. All of these fantasies are, of course, normal enough. But notice this: They keep you from dealing effectively with reality. Walter needs to learn to become more assertive with his wife. You need to let your boss know that you think your work is competent in a convincing, nonhostile way. If you get an F on a test, you need to acquire better study skills. And if you get a big tax bill, you need to develop a plan for paying it. A passing fantasy is harmless. But often it can interfere with effective action. If it is soothing enough to your ego, you will do nothing. So be aware of your tendency to employ passive fantasy as an ego defense. And don't get addicted to your fantasy life as if it offers any sort of solution.

You can, however, use fantasy in a constructive way. Almost all accomplishments were at first dreams. Kerry I. wanted to become an attorney. He watched a lot of Perry Mason shows. He often fantasized himself sitting in an office, interviewing clients, and presenting cases. His rich fantasy life was his way of creating a goal for himself. And he eventually became a successful attorney in real life. Often what you can visualize and imagine in your future can become a self-fulfilling prophecy.

When the odds are really against you and you can actually do nothing at all to change a situation, then fantasy can also be a constructive mental process. Frank W. Abagnale, author of *Catch Me If You Can*, was convicted of check fraud and was confined to a French prison. According to Abagnale, he lived for five months in a sort of dungeon without light or toilet facilities. He writes, "I think that I actually would have gone mad and died a lunatic in Perpignan prison had it not been for my vivid imagination. The creative ability that had enabled me to concoct the brilliant swindles I perpetrated over the years, and which had resulted in my present plight, now served as a lifeguard." In his voluntary fantasies, Abagnale saw himself as an airline pilot surrounded by glamorous stewardesses, as a hero, a tour bus driver, a famous surgeon, a movie director, and a Nobel Prize–winning author. It is clear that Abagnale used fantasy in a constructive way.

---

### MASTER STRATEGY 11

### Change your ego defense mechanisms from emotional liabilities into life-enhancing assets.

Although defense mechanisms arise from an unconscious level, they contain a conscious element. If you are reflective and thoughtful, you can catch yourself in the act. You can think, "Who's kidding whom?" And this question will often help you see that you are kidding yourself. The kind of self-deception that takes place when you use defense mechanisms in passive, self-defeating ways will aggravate your neurosis. And you are not likely to deal with your real-life problems in effective ways.

On the other hand, if you use defense mechanisms in positive, constructive ways, they can become mental forces that will help you survive and cope with life. This chapter has presented ways in which you can (1) avoid self-defeating defensive patterns and (2) employ constructive ones.

---

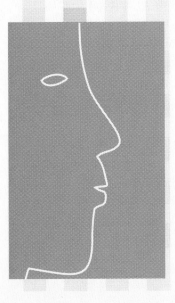

**Chapter 12**

# Even Freud Was Neurotic: Putting His Ideas to Work for You

**Yes, it's true.** Even Freud was neurotic. Freud, the fountainhead of modern psychotherapy, the famous scientist, and a maker and shaker of modern thought was a person who had his share of emotional problems.

The fact that Freud was neurotic undermines his credibility for some people. They make remarks such as, "Freud was crazy. Why pay any attention to what he says?"

In the first place, Freud was definitely *not* crazy. The informal word *crazy* suggests a state of psychosis, a delusional condition in which one is out of touch with reality. There is nothing in Freud's life history to suggest that he was at any time psychotic. To say that he was neurotic is to say that he was a troubled person. Chapter 3 explained the concept of neurosis, and you will recall that a core of anxiety characterizes neurosis. Also, neurotic persons tend to have problems with depression and anger. There are, of course, other aspects to the neurotic syndrome.

In the second place, let's consider why we should pay attention to what Freud has to say. The fact that he was neurotic should not undermine his credibility at all. Carl Jung, one of Freud's early colleagues said, "Only the wounded healer can heal." This statement, considering my work in counseling and psychotherapy, has always impressed me. I have been able to help compulsive eaters because I myself was once 70 pounds overweight. Although I have been at a more or less normal weight for many years, I still think of myself as a recovering compulsive eater, not a recovered one. I still have to think about what I do, remain alert to my eating tendencies, and not take anything for granted.

It is well known that some of the best counselors for alcoholics and drug addicts are recovering alcoholics and recovering drug addicts. The fact that Freud was a troubled person only means that with his intelligence and unusual abilities he was able to help himself and others. Being neurotic, he had the empathy and understanding that is required to be an effective psychotherapist.

## Freud's Life and Career

The two most famous thinkers of the twentieth century were Albert Einstein and Sigmund Freud. Einstein investigated the outer universe, the world outside the self. Freud investigated the inner universe, the domain of the mind.

Sigmund Freud was born in 1856 and died in 1939. He had eighty-three long years to accomplish his life's work, the establishment of psychoanalysis as both a school of psychology and a system of psychotherapy. He lived and worked primarily in Vienna, Austria, and he published more than twenty books on psychoanalysis. A number of them, including *The Interpretation of Dreams* and *The Psychopathology of Everyday Life,* are addressed not only to professionals but also to the general reader.

Raised in a poor family with several brothers and sisters, Freud was the firstborn, and his mother doted on him all his life. She called him her "Golden Siggy" and expected great things of him. He credits much of his accomplishment to her constant belief in his superior abilities. Freud derived the notion that there is an Oedipus complex, that some children can have an erotic attraction to a parent, from his memories of his early relationship with his mother as well as from some of the revelations of his patients. If Freud had Oedipal feelings, though, they were well repressed and well controlled. He was devoted to his mother well into her old age, and he was a stable married man with children of his own.

Freud was inspired to pursue science as a vocation after hearing a presentation of the poem "Nature" by the German author Johann Wolfgang von Goethe. Freud's initial interest was in biology, and he did significant work as a graduate student on the gonads of eels. He was advised against an academic career as a biologist by one of his professors, Ernst Brücke, who reluctantly informed Freud that he would have no future at the university level because he was Jewish.

Freud instead became a medical doctor and specialized in neurology. He studied under Martin Charcot in France, at that time the greatest neurologist in Europe. Working with Charcot, Freud learned that many people who seem to have a neurological illness are actually suffering from emotional conflicts and have convinced themselves that they have an organic problem. Charcot was able to demonstrate that under deep hypnosis some people who thought they could not see, or walk, or who believed a hand or arm was numb could in fact see, walk, and feel pain. This self-induced pseudoneurological illness was called *hysteria*.

Once Freud married and established his own medical practice, he became friends with a highly respected physician named Josef Breuer. Breuer had a patient known as Anna O. in the psychoanalytic literature. She suffered from hysteria, and Breuer found that he could alleviate her symptoms with hypnosis. Breuer and Anna discovered that just talking about her problems, often under hypnosis, had a profound beneficial effect. Anna nicknamed this process "chimney sweeping." It was one of the first examples of what came to be known as "the talking cure" or psychoanalysis.

Freud never saw Anna, but he also had patients suffering from hysteria. He tried Breuer's approach with good results and encouraged Breuer to publish their results together. Breuer eventually agreed to write a book with Freud. Titled *Studies in Hysteria*, it appeared in 1895 and is the first publication in psychoanalysis.

Breuer and Freud ceased to work together, and for about fifteen years Freud worked alone. He referred to this period as a time of "splendid isolation," seeing himself as a lonely pioneer. In time he attracted colleagues who were also interested in psychoanalysis. Carl Jung, a psychiatrist from Switzerland, read *The Interpretation of Dreams*, published in 1900, and became one of Freud's associates. The same book also attracted that attention of Alfred Adler, a Viennese ophthalmologist, and he joined Freud's growing circle of advocates. Freud, Jung, and Adler are considered to be the principal founders of modern psychotherapy. Eventually both men drifted away from Freud, primarily because of disagreements over psychological theory.

In 1909 Granville Stanley Hall, president of Clark University (Worcester, Massachusetts), invited Freud and Jung to the United States to give a series of lectures on psychoanalysis. Freud credited these lectures as a landmark moment that helped establish the credibility of psychoanalysis. The International Psychoanalytic Association was established in 1910. By the 1920s Freud was famous, and psychoanalysis had become a widely used method of therapy.

In 1938, responding to international pressure, the Nazi government gave Freud permission to emigrate from Austria to England. This was a rare exception because Freud was Jewish. He spent the remainder of his life in England, dying in 1939.

## Putting Freud's Ideas to Work

Usually when people think of psychoanalysis, they think of going to a psychiatrist or a psychologist who practices this kind of therapy. More than one movie has portrayed a patient reclining on a couch, making free associations or telling about a dream. However, you don't have to think about Freud's ideas in a strictly professional setting. They imply self-applications, and you can put them to work without spending time on a psychiatrist's couch. This section presents self-directed psychological strategies based on psychoanalytic theory. They are designed to help you live at greater peace with your neurosis.

### *Self-Analysis*

🔦

### Make a self-analysis.

Freud was never analyzed by anyone other than himself. He never went to a therapist and reclined on a couch. In a way, this is logical. Who can help the Master? Who was competent to analyze the father of psychoanalysis? The obvious answer is that there was no one who could do the job for Freud that he did for others.

Freud's self-analysis spanned a ten-year period. During this time he kept a nearly daily record of his free associations (or random thoughts), dreams, speech errors, and various behavioral errors. He interpreted them in terms of his understanding of the human personality. Material that was formerly buried at an unconscious level became accessible at a conscious, rational level. Freud gained insight into the meaning of early childhood memories. He also discovered forbidden wishes of either a sexual or aggressive nature. Although we really can't say that he "cured" himself of his neurosis, he found practical ways to live with himself and his emotional problems. He became a more effective person and a better therapist.

Within limits, you can do some of what Freud did for himself. You can make a self-analysis. This procedure has already been explained and described in some detail in Chapter 11 under the subheading "Repression." Turn back to that chapter to review ways to conduct a written self-analysis.

### The Importance of Dreams

Use Freud's principles to interpret your dreams.

Freud said that dreams are the "royal road to the unconscious." Before Freud came on the scene, dreams were regarded in a variety of ways. Many ancient cultures assumed that dreams were visits from the gods, that they were prophetic in nature, giving a glimpse of the future. Other traditions believed that a dream is a spiritual voyage the soul makes, leaving the body during sleep.

According to Freud, dreams are part of the natural mental processes of the personality; they reveal what is repressed at an unconscious level. Freud stated that dreams, particularly those of neurotic persons, usually have two levels. The *manifest level* of a dream is what is actually dreamed. It is the story and images that are consciously remembered when the dreamer awakens. The *latent level* of a dream is what the dream means. The meaning is usually contained within a forbidden wish. The reason that the dream appears in an often confused and strange form is that a kind of censorship is being exercised by the defense mechanism of repression. The dream itself is a kind of "leakage" or escape of repressed material from the unconscious level to the conscious one. During sleep, the internal censor is somewhat relaxed and not quite as vigilant as during wakefulness.

If you want to interpret your dreams in order to gain greater insight into the more profound levels of your personality, you first have to "capture" your dreams. Many people say that they can't remember their dreams, or they only remember small fragments. Keep a notepad on a bedside table or in the bathroom. When you awaken during the night, you often have just had a dream. This is the time when it is most vivid. Jot down immediately whatever you remember. When you have the opportunity later to write in your self-analysis journal, explore your dream in terms of Freud's distinction between the manifest and the latent content. Ask yourself what the dream might be telling you about your repressed emotional life. What forbidden wish does it seem to disclose? Use free association to unlock this understanding as you would with repression in general.

Sharon H. made the following interpretation of one of her recurrent dreams:

More than once I dreamed I was on a desert island, far away from home. The sky was blue, I had plenty to eat, and there were no people around. I felt content and at peace. My free associations brought me to the conclusion that the dream was one of escape. That seems pretty obvious, of course. But the thing I wasn't facing at first was that I wanted to escape from my marriage. I had recognized for some time at some level that my marriage was unhappy and I wanted out. But I was a traditional woman. I not only didn't want to admit failure, I also felt guilty for wanting to be done with my husband. The dream told me the truth. My forbidden wish was to leave him. At this point I'm not sure if I want to work on my marriage, if there is any hope, or if I really, realistically want to end it. But at least I know that at some sort of basic emotional level the wish is there, and it helps me to think clearly about what I want to do because I am dealing with something I know about myself, not some obscure muddle.

Shane I. made the following interpretation of one of his dreams:

I dreamed I was walking down a long white corridor with many doors. I liked being there. Suddenly there seemed to be a lot of hustle and bustle. And then there were people in pain. I was able to calm them down. It was a good feeling. Then I abruptly woke up. My random associations to the dream led me to the conclusion that the place I was dreaming about was a hospital. My forbidden wish is that I want to go into the medical profession. I've always been attracted to the art of healing. The wish is "forbidden" because I think, at least at a conscious level, that it's too late. I'm forty-three years old, have three children, and am a certified public accountant. I probably won't make the switch, drop everything, and go to medical school. But I *can* work as a volunteer, acquire some counseling skills, and meet the need expressed in my forbidden wish in a way that is a compromise between the wishful life and the realistic life.

### Slips of the Tongue

Use Freud's principles to interpret your slips of the tongue, minor accidents, and everyday blunders.

One of Freud's most readable books is *The Psychopathology of Everyday Life*. In this book Freud asserted that slips of the tongue and other blunders provide glimpses of unconscious motives. Blaine S. was in bed with his wife around midnight. The lights were off. He said, "Before I go to sleep, I want to kill you tonight."

His wife, startled, sat up in bed, turned on a light, and asked, "What did you mean by that?"

He replied, "Nothing. I meant to say I want to kiss you tonight."

She stared at him, uncertain. "I don't get it."

He said, "Can't a guy make a mistake? It was an innocent thing. I just wanted to kiss you good night."

Blaine and his wife had been arguing most of the evening. He was building up a load of resentment. The slip of the tongue is an expression of hostility. No, Blaine doesn't actually want to kill his wife. But the primitive id, the unsocialized infant within the personality, entertains the idea. Blaine can use his slip to gain greater insight into his hidden self.

This question always arises at an academic level in a psychology class: Do all slips of the tongue mean something? Or are some of them just innocent errors? Freud seemed to think that just about all slips of the tongue provided a window onto unconscious motives. Today's thinking suggests that some slips have more to do with conflicting habits than with unconscious motives. For example, let's say that someone asks you for your phone number. You answer, "Area code 606-743-4401." You hesitate. "What am I saying? It's area code 702-783-5329." Why did you make the error? In this case, assume that you moved to a new residence just three weeks ago. When asked for your phone number, you answer out of habit with the number at your old residence. The habit of using your old number takes temporary priority over using your new number. Such a slip is called a Watsonian slip in honor of John B. Watson, a major learning theorist and the father of behaviorism.

On the other hand, the kind of slip that Blaine made hardly seems Watsonian. He is much more used to saying, "I want to kiss you" than "I want to kill you." Blaine's slip does appear to reveal unconscious hostility. Consequently, this kind of slip is called a Freudian slip in honor of Freud's emphasis on the importance of unconscious motives.

It is not only slips of the tongue that reveal unconscious motives. Such slips are only one of a group of errors that have a similar theme. Alan C. worked as a carpenter. He laughed that he was a klutz. He was always banging his thumb with a hammer, bumping into things, and once sawed off the tip of his index finger. Accident-prone, he recognized that something was wrong. Facing inner reality, he discovered that at an unconscious level he wanted to make a new start and find a different career field. In time, Alan became a high school history teacher.

Look at your errors, whatever they may be, and ask yourself what unconscious motives they suggest. Forbidden wishes usually reside behind what Freud called the psychopathology of everyday life. If you can recognize and identify an unconscious motive, it will cease to exercise an involuntary, negative effect on your life. You can think about it in the light of reason. You can evaluate it in terms of reality.

### An Active Determinism

Use the deterministic outlook of psychoanalysis to find your own direction in life.

Freud was a strict psychological determinist. He believed that we live in a completely cause-and-effect universe, and that this principle is also always at work in the human mind. That is why he saw as meaningful dreams, slips of the tongue, and other behaviors that are often discounted. To Freud, everything was a piece of the mental jigsaw puzzle.

Unfortunately, if misinterpreted, the deterministic outlook can induce despair. One feels helpless in a universe that one did not make. The general outlook is that "I can't help what I do today because of what happened to me in the past." The attitude is that of a victim, a pawn of fate.

You will recall that one of the self-directed strategies recommended in Chapter 6 was *Affirm the existence of your free will*. This strategy is in opposition to the deterministic outlook. At a strict philosophical level, Freud rejected the existence of free will. Nonetheless, it is clear that everything he did at a professional level was designed to set individuals free from the adverse influence of unfortunate past events. Yes, Freud saw us as shaped by experiences. But the strategies of psychoanalysis are designed to be working tools that set you free from the prison created by the past. You use determinism against itself. You fight fire with fire. In the end, this approach, like the assertion of free will, helps you find your autonomy. It helps you become the self-directed person you seek to be.

A passive determinism is not much more than a "poor me" attitude. An active determinism asserts that you can use the cause-and-effect principle to rise above the fate that was imposed upon you against your will. Freud did it. In spite of his neurosis, he was a highly autonomous person, a person in charge of his own life. Allow Freud to be a role model for you. Affirm that by understanding the chain of cause and effect in your life, you can also break the chain.

### Facing Life Head-On

🌡

#### Seek it, and you will find your existential courage.

What is *existential courage?* It is the courage *to be,* to face life squarely. It is the psychological attitude that you will prevail, that you will be a survivor, come what may. I place this viewpoint squarely in the camp of Freud's thought because he provides an outstanding example of what is meant by existential courage. In his youth he fought poverty and the general discrimination against Jewish persons to become a physician and an eminent neurologist. In his maturity he worked alone for a number of years, willing to endure the rejection of the psychiatric establishment, in order to put forth the ideas that eventually became psychoanalysis. He kept writing his books even when, at first, *The Interpretation of Dreams,* a book he considered his masterpiece, sold dismally.

In his old age, he endured for many years the pain and suffering associated with cancer of the mouth. Nonetheless, he kept working and seeing patients.

But how do you, like Freud, find your existential courage? You *seek* it. If you do, if you genuinely look for it, you will *find* it. Because it is there. It is part and parcel of your being. It is a built-in component of the self. Let's say that there is a 1-pound bag of sugar in your pantry. It really is there. If you look for it, look with conviction, you will find it, won't you? You can't help but find it. The same thing is true about your existential courage. It's there. Maybe it's buried or hidden, just as the bag of sugar may be behind a can of coffee. But if you remove the obstacles, what you are looking for can be found.

If you look for the strength to carry on, if you seek your existential courage, you will discover it.

## MASTER STRATEGY 12

### Think about your life in psychodynamic terms.

The word *psychodynamic* refers to the fact that the inner world, the world of the self, is a field of opposing forces. The term has its roots in Freud's psychoanalysis. In a practical sense, thinking about your life in psychodynamic terms suggests that you recognize the complexity of your personal nature. There are pushes and pulls within you. There are forbidden wishes that are in conflict with moral injunctions. It is a good idea to come to terms with your conflicts. If you can't completely end the civil war within yourself, you can reduce the intensity of the battle. This chapter, inspired by Freud's teachings, has provided some psychological strategies that will help you.

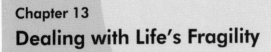

Chapter 13
# Dealing with Life's Fragility

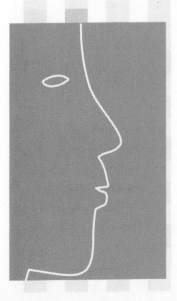

**To some extent,** it is natural to be neurotic. This is because you can think and reflect on life itself.

When you do reflect on life, it becomes obvious that it is fragile, that it can end at any time in unexpected ways. Or, its quality can be destroyed by an accident or an illness. Shawna M., a young mother with two children, told me, "I don't feel the world is a solid thing. To me, it's not an object like a rock. It's more like a soap bubble, a bubble that can burst at any moment. I look around me and when I see my husband, my home, my children, my life, and my presently good health I feel that it can just end at any time—burst apart like a soap bubble. I know it's the wrong attitude, an outlook that makes me constantly nervous and tense. But I don't know what to do about it."

The kind of anxiety that Shawna is talking about is called *existential anxiety*. It is the fear of death and disability. In and of itself existential anxiety is not abnormal. It is impossible for a human being to shake such anxiety completely. I doubt that an ant or a shark experiences existential anxiety. They live and die, struggle and eat, but they aren't built in such a way that they can dwell on the risks of their existence. In fact, the more you can think and imagine possibilities, the more likely you are to suffer from existential anxiety.

There are unimaginative, nonreflective people who live blissfully like the animals. They rush through life as if they were bulls, full of energy and commitment, without a moment's thought devoted to what an unlikely and unstable structure existence is. When you talk about risks and dangers, they look at you with uncomprehending eyes. They can't imagine that their own life can possibly end. Incidentally, don't think of such people as courageous. They are basically foolhardy. A courageous person is one who sees the dangers, experiences fear, and copes with his or her emotions in order to keep on functioning. In reading this book, in making an effort to apply its self-directed strategies, you are being courageous.

Existential anxiety, as already indicated, is not abnormal. However, if you suffer from *chronic* existential anxiety, the kind Shawna described, then you have an *existential neurosis*. You can't get completely rid of existential anxiety. It comes and goes like the wind. It's unpleasant when you experience it, but the impression passes, and you carry on. If, on the other hand, you are living with existential anxiety on a daily basis, you want to do something about it. And this chapter will give you some tools that will help you cope.

## Understanding Existentialism

Before we proceed, it's a good idea to explain a little about the philosophy known as existentialism. *Existentialism* is the point of view that life as it is actually experienced on a day-to-day basis by the individual is far more important than any so-called objective description, be it scientific or philosophical. Let's say that you have just awakened from a dream. It just so happens that you are a subject participating in sleep research. You casually mention to the scientist in charge that you just had a dream. You are told that you didn't have a dream because no rapid-eye-movement (REM) episodes were associated with the time period in question. Also, your electroencephalogram (EEG) shows a lot of slow delta waves. These are associated with deep sleep, a kind of sleep that doesn't produce dreams. Who's right? The scientist or you? If you have any common sense at all, you will believe yourself. You will trust your experience, not an objective, external analysis. This is an existential approach. (Incidentally, sleep research does support the general idea that a few dreams of a very murky nature, dreams without sharp imagery, can take place during deep sleep.)

Let's apply the existential way of thinking to something more profound than whether you actually had a dream. Let's assume that you believe in your free will. You have confidence that you have the power of choice. A behaviorist such as B. F. Skinner says that you don't. He explains that everything is cause and effect. As an organism, you live in a physical universe, and your body is a part of that universe. According to this view, what you call your mind is just the activity of the brain and the nervous system, the excitation and inhibition of neurons associated with the activity of chemical messengers. This process combined with your learning history makes you the person you are. Your sense of freedom and mine is just a false perception, a kind of mass delusion of the human race. It has no reality at all. In some ways, this argument is powerful and compelling.

And yet, you *feel* free. Existentialism says not to allow logic to take precedence over your experience. You are in direct contact with your freedom. You know you are free the way you know that you walk and talk and think. It is a given of your conscious mind. Again, if you have any common sense, you will not doubt that you have free will, or at least the potential for free will.

### Kierkegaard's Search

The father of existentialism is usually said to be the nineteenth-century Danish philosopher Søren Kierkegaard. Kierkegaard had extensive training in classical philosophy. He noted that all of his academic knowledge didn't help him deal with his personal problems, particularly the problem of existential anxiety. And he had a bad case. Two of his books are called *Fear and Trembling* and *The Concept of Dread*. He tried to work out a philosophy of life that would help him survive, to be able to walk the rocky road of existence. It has to be admitted that he made only a so-so job of his own life. He was on-again/off-again about marrying a particular woman, and in the end he never did marry her. He spent most of his large inheritance self-publishing books that sold poorly, and he died at the age of forty-two.

Nonetheless, Kierkegaard is considered an existential pioneer. He pointed the way toward a psychological world that is less plagued with existential anxiety. He emphasized the importance of thinking for yourself, and he stressed that the individual is unique. He said that he wanted engraved on his tombstone only these words: The Individual.

### Sartre's Self-Awareness

The most influential existentialist of the twentieth century was the French philosopher and novelist Jean-Paul Sartre. A survivor of both World War I and World War II, he encountered the fragility of existence head-on. His greatest work,

*Being and Nothingness,* sets forth the essence of modern existential philosophy. He contended that our way of being in the world is different than the kind of being possessed by rocks and animals. They have "being-in-itself," meaning that they exist without self-awareness. We have "being-for-itself," meaning that we exist with self-awareness. This self-awareness is, of course, what induces existential anxiety. However, this same self-awareness also makes it possible for us to reduce the intensity of an agonizing existential anxiety.

Sartre asserts that we have freedom of the will, intelligence, memory, the power to imagine the future, self-awareness, and existential courage. We may lose sight of these psychological possessions, but they are never gone. They are a part of us just like our fingers, our hair, and our eyes. Our will and related psychological faculties are our powers. They make it possible for us to cope with existential anxiety, and they reduce the emotional suffering associated with the very risk of being alive.

## Coping with Existential Anxiety

Let us now identify specific self-directed strategies that will help you cope with existential anxiety. Let's put to work the kind of faculties identified by Kierkegaard and Sartre. Think of your will, intelligence, memory, imagination, self-awareness, and existential courage as tools in a mental toolbox. They are there waiting to be used. Maybe they're getting rusty, just like real tools. But if you take them out and put them to work, they will be self-sharpening, and you will find that little by little the job of coping with existential anxiety gets somewhat easier.

The following self-directed strategies automatically call on your psychological tools, the very real powers of your mind.

### Acting As If the Future Were Real

🔦

#### Recognize that we live in an as-if world.

Shawna M.'s observation that we live in a kind of soap bubble is, unfortunately, a profound truth of existence. Life as we know it may pop and go to pieces at any moment. Ordinary language trains us to think and act as if the future were real. We say, "I'll see you tomorrow." Or, we say, "Next week I'll take a trip." Or, we say, "This summer I'm going to catch up on my reading." When you are free from existential anxiety, you live in a psychological world that is rich with future.

But when you recognize that ordinary language usage doesn't reflect reality—that, in fact, you could die at any moment—you are flooded with existential anxiety. And this is not foolishness. It is reality. Every day people die or are badly injured in auto accidents. Planes frequently crash. Dreaded illnesses become realities when a physician makes a diagnosis. If you are acutely aware of these kinds of possibilities, you are living in an as-if world. You know that the future as you imagine it doesn't really exist—not yet—but you decide to act as if it does.

It may seem odd that the recommended strategy here is to recognize that we live in an as-if world. It would appear that the wise thing to do is to deny this fact, to repress it, to get rid of it. Unfortunately, if you are already aware of the fragility of existence, denial of this particular reality will only aggravate your existential neurosis. The effort to deny is stressful. And it won't be successful. At a shadow level, your unconscious mind will keep whispering to you, "It's a dangerous world out there. Anything can happen. You hang by a thread."

No, the only thing you can do if you are disposed in the direction of an existential neurosis is to face facts, stop denying reality. Admit that you and I, all of us, live in an as-if world. Say to yourself, "The future is not real, but I will act as if it were." Say to yourself, "I don't know what will happen tomorrow, but I will act as if I do." Say to yourself, "I will live and work as if tomorrow were real." If the as-if is all you have to work with, then turn it into your makeshift foundation. Employ your intelligence to see reality as it is. And employ your existential courage to carry on.

### Facing Death

Think of your biological death as an event of only modest importance.

The fear of death resides at the very core of existential anxiety. That is why it is important to start looking at it not as a big, big deal, but as a somewhat inconsequential event.

"Wait a minute," you may be saying. "A somewhat inconsequential event! What could be more consequential than death?"

A reasonable question, to be sure. However, it all depends on how you look at, and learn to accept, the meaning of death.

Written in the nineteenth century, Leo Tolstoy's short novel *The Death of Ivan Ilyich* vividly portrays the fear of death and its conquest. The story reflects the author's own concerns. One of those people who went through life like a bull with no thought of either death or the as-if quality of existence, Ivan is brought up short by a diagnosis of cancer.

A self-important person, a court judge, Ivan finds it hard to accept that life will go on for others after he is gone, that his death will make only a ripple. Toward the end of his life, he grows in psychological maturity and takes a larger view. He recognizes that death is a part of a natural process, and he is able to accept it with peace of mind.

You probably have one of two beliefs. First, you may believe in the reality of the afterlife. You are convinced that your soul is immortal; that your personal self transcends biological death and continues to be conscious and remember the past after your body is left behind.

Second, you may believe that death is oblivion. The ego is blotted out. You are pretty sure that when you die, it really is The End. Using the existential language of Sartre, you see death as the end of Being and the beginning of Nothingness.

Let's say that you favor the first alternative. For you, death is really an event of only modest importance. It is not an ending, but a doorway into another kind of life, a life in which you will be reunited with friends and loved ones. In this second life, you will experience only joy. And there will be no pain. If you accept the first alternative, clearly there is nothing to fear.

On the other hand, let's say that you favor the second alternative. For you, death is really a nonevent because *you can't experience it*. You can experience that you're about to die or the pain of an illness or injury, but you can't experience death itself because there is no ego, no personality, to experience the death. You can experience everything up to the threshold of death, but when death comes there is no vision, no hearing, no awareness at all. In short, when you're dead, you don't know you're dead. From an existential point of view, life is immortal because all that you can ever experience is life itself. For you, the living personality, the circle of life is never closed.

Both alternatives, from a psychological point of view, reduce your biological death to an event of modest importance. Accepting this mental attitude will help you enjoy life because it will reduce the level of your existential anxiety.

### Growing in Confidence

🕯

**Believe in your own emotional resourcefulness.**

Have confidence that you will be able to cope with whatever fate hands you. You have your doubts about yourself. You wonder if you can keep going, if you have what it takes to deal with whatever is in store for you. Your neurotic imagination often presents you with vivid fantasies of personal disasters. And you're afraid that you won't be able to cope. But look back at your past. Somehow you have managed, haven't you? You didn't always make the best choices. You made mistakes. But you muddled through somehow. In the same way that you've managed to muddle through until now, you'll be able to survive tomorrow. In fact, you'll probably do better than you've done in the past. You've been learning. Life is a great teacher. And it is a well-known psychological phenomenon that people not only learn; they *learn to learn*. So as you get older, it will get easier because you learn to become more effective. You grow in wisdom. And the self-directed strategies presented in this book should also be of significant help.

## *Making Your Intelligence Work for You*

🔔

### Fight psychological fire with psychological fire.

It is the "fire" of your intelligence that causes existential anxiety. As already suggested, persons who are not bright and reflective, who do not imagine possibilities, suffer from little or no existential anxiety. The best way to cope with the negative effects of your own intelligence is to apply that same intelligence to take a larger view of life. Using your intelligence to cope with intelligence itself suggests that you have a *metaintelligence*, or intelligence above and beyond ordinary intelligence.

It is the gloom and doom caused by ordinary intelligence that induces existential anxiety. You are all too aware of the risks and dangers of life. You know you live in an as-if world. Sometimes you feel you hang by a thread. When you employ ordinary intelligence, you are both aware and imaginative about life, but you are not reflective and analytical about your own thought processes. You are just letting them flow in a reactive, noncritical way. Your thinking seems right just because it's your thinking.

On the other hand, when you employ metaintelligence, you reflect on your own thought processes. You ask yourself questions. You challenge the ideas and images that are being fed to you by ordinary intelligence.

Brian C. is a real estate broker. He was wealthy in his early thirties. Married with three children, he says, "I used to suffer from severe existential anxiety. I had a full-blown existential neurosis. I imagined that I could lose all of my assets at any time if the real estate bubble burst. I thought I was living a good life, but on borrowed time. My father died in his late forties of a heart attack. I felt that I could be plunged into the pit of nonbeing at any time. I reacted by living the fast life. I gambled heavily in Las Vegas. I became a workaholic. I burned the candle at both ends. Yes, and I got a girlfriend on the side. It nearly destroyed my marriage. I used to say and really believed, 'Live today; for tomorrow we may die.' Then I was introduced by a clinical psychologist to a short essay by O. Hobart Mowrer, a former president of the American Psychological Association.

"Mowrer, in counseling wayward adolescents, often heard them say something along the lines that we should live today because we might die tomorrow. Mowrer's answer was, 'That's right. But we usually don't die tomorrow.' That hit me hard. Yes, we can die tomorrow. *But we usually don't.* This was a turning point for me. I began to look upon life as being open with possibilities. Yes, I might die young. But I might not. I began to feel better and the level of my existential anxiety dropped."

Brian has learned to fight psychological fire with psychological fire. He is using metaintelligence to dampen the emotional blaze induced by ordinary intelligence.

### A Long Life to Live

🍏

**Tell yourself that in spite of all its dangers, life will probably be long.**

Today's life expectancy at birth is approximately seventy-four years. This is, of course, the expectancy for infants, not adults, a fact that many people fail to recognize. If you are— let's say—thirty-five years old, your actual expectancy is about seventy-six years. If you are fifty years old, your actual expectancy is about seventy-eight years. This is because, from a statistical viewpoint, you pick up the expectancy of people who have died before you.

The odds are in your favor. It is probable that you will live even longer than these figures suggest. This is because you are neurotic. And, on the whole, neurotic people tend to be more cautious than others. They watch their health because of their hypochondriacal tendencies (see Chapter 9). Being somewhat obsessive and phobic, neurotics try to avoid danger. So maybe you can add a few years to the numbers cited here.

Like Freud, Carl Jung, one of the founders of modern psychotherapy, suffered from a neurosis. He combated his own existential anxiety by deliberately imagining a long life for himself. He said that in his youth he felt old age in his bones. He fully recognized that we live in an as-if world. But he decided that his own as-if world would be constructed in such a way that it contained longevity. Born in 1875, he died in 1961 at the age of eighty-six.

### Appreciating What Life Offers

🔌

**Recognize the positive payoff of existential anxiety.**

Existential anxiety is uncomfortable. It is not pleasant to feel that existence is like a soap bubble. And you do want to seek ways to diminish this kind of anxiety by using self-directed strategies such as those described in this chapter. Nonetheless, you should also realize that existential anxiety has a positive payoff. Wrapped in its brown outer paper is a gift of real importance. This is the gift of appreciation.

Existential anxiety gives us a profound appreciation for the value of life. The fact that all of *this,* everything you see and hear, can be snatched away at any instant intensifies your awareness of the beauty of the world, of the laughter of children, of the precious quality of real love.

An ant can't experience existential anxiety. Nor can it appreciate the value of life. Without reflection and an awareness of the fragility of existence, there cannot be a sense of wonder and exaltation that we exist at all. Human beings who take life completely for granted, who can't imagine nonexistence, cannot possibly have the appreciation for life that you have. A valued object is all the more precious when you realize that it can be lost. Similarly, the process of living acquires a sharper, more vivid quality when you are reminded that the process won't go on forever.

Roxanne E. is a forty-four-year-old pharmacist. She recently had major surgery to remove a tumor on a kidney. She says, "I was given a total anesthetic for my surgery. As I was rolled on the gurney into the operating room, I was overcome with the feeling that I might lose consciousness not for the relatively brief period of surgery, but forever. My heart began to pound as I realized that maybe this was it. I am one of those people who regard death as oblivion. And then somehow I was able to accept that I might die. I remember thinking, as they say in Italy, '*Che sara, sara,*' or, 'What will be, will be.' When I came out of my unconscious state, back to the world, I remember thinking, 'If that was anything like death, it was nothing to be afraid of.' Then I saw a picture on the wall of the recovery room. It was just an inexpensive print of birds. But they seemed indescribably beautiful. Tears came into my eyes. Then my husband joined me. The concern on his face and the love in his eyes touched my heart in a way that it had not been touched in years. I think he was surprised by how tightly I squeezed his hand."

Roxanne's experience clearly demonstrates that a close call with death enhances our appreciation for that which life has to offer.

Naturally, you don't want to go around experiencing existential anxiety all of the time. What you want to get rid of is this kind of chronic anxiety, the kind that defines an existential neurosis. On the other hand, occasional pangs of existential anxiety are not all bad. They bring out the richness and fullness of life. They show us that life is not to be taken for granted.

## Finding Courage

### ♥

**Reaffirm the reality of your existential courage.**

You will recall that the concept of existential courage was introduced earlier in association with Freud's thought (see Chapter 12). I asserted that if you seek your courage, you will find it. You need existential courage to cope with existential anxiety. Roxanne found it when she faced major surgery.

Shawna M., introduced in the opening of this chapter, found her existential courage in the process of psychotherapy. You will recall that Shawna said, "I don't feel the world is a solid thing. To me, it's not an object like a rock. It's more like a soap bubble, a bubble that can burst at any moment." Now she says, "I haven't gotten rid of the feeling that everything can vanish at any moment. But it's not with me all of the time. It comes and goes, mostly goes. When the sensation does make an appearance, when it intrudes, I face it squarely. I don't mentally try to run away from it. I don't try to deny that it's there or wish that it would go away. I tell myself that I have the courage to go on, that I'm a survivor, and I find the courage I'm looking for. I remember a line from the musical play, *The King and I*. The line is in the song, 'Whistle a Happy Tune.' The line says that you may be as brave as you make-believe you are. The lesson seems to be that by acting brave you become brave. I have found that this is so."

### MASTER STRATEGY 13

*Realize that we can learn to live relatively unafraid in a world we never made.*

Existential philosophers speak of the *thrown* quality of existence. This means that we are, in a sense, thrown into this world against our will. It's a world we did not make. Perhaps if we had any say in the matter, we would have designed a different, better world. But here we are. The image comes to mind of the shipwrecked central character in Daniel Defoe's eighteenth-century novel, *Robinson Crusoe*. (The novel is based on the actual adventures of Alexander Selkirk, a Scottish sailor). He chose to work at survival, and survive he did. You were thrown onto this planet at this moment in time in the same way that Robinson was tossed by the sea onto his island. Robinson grew fairly secure on his island as his survival skills improved. Similarly, you can grow fairly secure in your corner of the world as your own survival skills improve.

I say that you can learn to live *relatively* unafraid. Being a thinking person, you can't rid yourself completely of existential anxiety. Nor do you need to. Remember once again that such anxiety has its own positive payoff. But you can learn to live without chronic existential anxiety, the kind of steady-state anxiety that corrodes the quality of life.

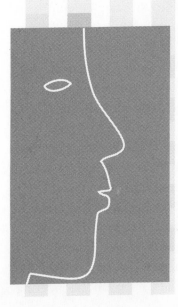

## Chapter 14
# Channel Your Neurosis into a Meaningful Life

**What is life** all about?

Why were you born?

Why are you living?

Tough questions. If you can't answer these questions to your own satisfaction, then you will suffer from an existential vacuum. An *existential vacuum* exists when life appears to have no value, no meaning, and no real purpose.

If an existential vacuum is chronic, then you are suffering from an *existential neurosis*. This kind of neurosis will interact with your everyday neurotic disposition and greatly aggravate your level of emotional distress. At the extreme, the combination of an existential neurosis and a neurotic personality will lead to a life of despair.

It is essential that you fill in the existential vacuum with meaning. Then it is possible to go on. It is not only essential to do this, it is within your power; both existentialism and humanistic psychology teach that this is so.

Perhaps you don't suffer from an existential neurosis. I hope so. However, many human beings either do or are skating on the thin ice of a borderline existential neurosis. If you sense that you're skating on thin psychological ice, this chapter will help you keep from breaking through and falling into the icy waters of psychological emptiness.

The truth is that it is a part of the human condition to face the challenge of meaning. Thinking, reflecting, and wondering automatically lead us from time to time to ask the question that introduced this chapter: What is life all about?

## Humanistic Psychology

The term *humanistic psychology* is basically self-explanatory. It is a psychology directed specifically toward human beings. It addresses that which is unique in us and probably not evident in animal behavior. The broad general themes of humanistic psychology point the way toward a meaningful life.

The father of humanistic psychology is Abraham Maslow. He died in 1970 at the age of sixty-two. Maslow's extremely influential teachings included the concept of self-actualization. *Self-actualization* is an inborn tendency to find ourselves, to become the persons we are meant to be. This is experienced as a psychological need to maximize our talents and potentialities. If a person can become self-actualizing, an important value has been met, and this will help that individual find meaning in life.

Maslow tells the story of one of his graduate students, a young woman who wanted to become a psychologist. It was the Great Depression of the 1930s, and she had dropped out of school to become a supervisor on an assembly line that produced chewing gum. She was discouraged and in a state of despair. She felt she couldn't quit her job because, although a single woman, she was the sole support of a rather large family. Maslow urged her, no matter how tired she was or how demanding her job, to take one graduate class a semester. In this way she would be self-actualizing. She would be working toward her goals and dreams. She followed Maslow's advice, and her sense of despair vanished.

At least three important points can be derived from the story. First, self-actualization is a human value; it is something worth doing. Second, the young woman's sense of despair was clearly existential, arising from the feeling that her job had no meaning and she couldn't become the person she was meant to be. Third, self-actualization is not an end state; it is a *process*. It is not the arrival at the goal that is required for the depression to lift, merely the awareness that the journey has started.

One of the outstanding contributors to humanistic psychology is the existential psychiatrist Viktor Frankl. Frankl died in 1997 at the age of ninety-two. His most famous book, *Man's Search for Meaning,* sets forth the system he called *logotherapy.* Logotherapy is both a philosophy of life and a system for helping troubled people. As a philosophy of life, logotherapy asserts that we have free will and that through the use of our will and intelligence, we can find a meaningful life. As a system for helping troubled people, logotherapy helps them overcome the emptiness of existence. Indeed, it was Frankl who coined the term *existential vacuum,* a concept defined earlier.

Frankl derived some of his ideas from his experiences in Nazi concentration camps during World War II. He discovered that even under the most adverse circumstances, it is possible to take a psychological stand against conditions, to avoid being defeated at an emotional level. In fact the original title of *Man's Search for Meaning* was *From Death Camp to Existentialism.* During his incarceration, Frankl found his meaning by continuing to function to the best of his ability as a healer. By giving whatever help and solace he could, he avoided the emotional nothingness of the existential vacuum.

Maslow's and Frankl's ideas, taken together, provide a powerful psychological antidote to the poison of *nihilism,* a point of view that denies the importance of all values, of everything that seems to make life worthwhile. The self-directed strategies that follow are informed and inspired by their teachings.

## Toward a Meaningful Life

Operating on the assumption that you are neurotic, you face a double challenge in your search for meaning. The anxiety and emotional conflict that you carry with you as part of your personality greatly aggravate any tendency you might have to think of life as pointless. It is far too easy to become cynical and to find the sorry side of almost everything. The aim of the psychological strategies presented in this section is to help you discover the pathway toward a meaningful life.

### *A Sense of Meaning*

🔦

**Reject the view that life is pointless and absurd.**

About five years ago Nicholas G., a forty-four-year-old horticulturist with a successful business, an attractive wife, and two bright children, told me, "'Life is a tale full of sound and fury, told by an idiot, signifying nothing.' I remember coming across this line in a play by Shakespeare when I was taking a high school English class. And it stuck. It seemed to be true in some way. And, now more than ever, I think that the whole thing's just one big joke. People talk about the meaning of life. They don't know what they're talking about."

One of the first things I told Nicholas was, "You must reject the view that life is pointless and absurd. This is known as nihilism. And it is the beginning of the road to nowhere. I can't prove that life is *not* absurd. But neither can you prove that it is. The fact of the matter is that if you start with the assumption that life has meaning, you are likely to discover that meaning. For human beings, it is next to impossible to live with any sense of personal satisfaction or desire to go forward in life without some sense of meaning."

This was a starting point for Nicholas. In spite of his statement, he yearned for meaning, as all of us do, and he listened. Today, after counseling and a substantial amount of reflection, he lives a meaningful life.

Reject nihilism. Look at life as potentially rich with significance. Make this the starting point of your own search for meaning.

### Finding Your Vocation

🍏

### Listen to the call of your life.

Jack London's most famous book was *The Call of the Wild*. It is about a dog named Buck who yearns to return to the wilderness and eventually does. Although it seems to be about a dog, the story is a metaphor for the author's own life. London had to obey his own call to become an adventurer and a writer. A bold man, full of energy and life, he overcame poverty and lack of connections to become at one time the most popular author in the United States. The theme of London's *The Call of the Wild* seems to be that you must discover the truth about your own inner nature. This will tell you what your calling in life is—your true vocation. And if you obey that call, you will find meaning in life.

It is interesting to note that the word *vocation* is derived from the Latin word *vox*, meaning voice. Originally, this meant that the voice of God was calling a person to become a priest or a nun. Today, the word has been generalized to have a more secular meaning. Nonetheless, if properly understood, a true vocation is something you were meant to do. Maslow writes about listening to one's inner impulse voices. You need to "listen" to your own inner nature. This will direct you toward your calling in life.

### Using Compulsions to Help You

🍂

**Direct your compulsive tendencies toward the pursuit of meaning.**

As the discovery of meaning is so important, here is one of life's arenas where your neurotic compulsive tendencies will be of real assistance. You will find that people who lead lives of high significance are often very single-minded in their search for meaning. Examples include the medical-missionary work of Albert Schweitzer, the merciful labors of Mother Teresa, the 1,000 patents of Thomas Alva Edison, the collected works of Sigmund Freud, and the many paintings of Pablo Picasso. You can say that these people were compulsive and neurotic. And you would probably be right. Also, you can say that they were full of zeal and dedication, and that these attributes made it possible for them to live lives that really counted. And you would also be right.

Your compulsive tendencies will supply the mental energy required to see long-term personal projects through to a successful conclusion.

## Leading a Full Life

💡

**Beware of putting all your eggs in one basket.**

The problem with the single-minded pursuit of one particular calling in life is that it can sometimes be destructive to personal relationships. Putting all of your eggs in the one basket of a particular identity or vocation has its own risks. As mentioned before, the life of the nineteenth-century painter Paul Gauguin provides a case in point. He abandoned his wife and children and finally settled in Tahiti. He died at the age of fifty-five, possibly of leprosy or syphilis. He left behind a set of important paintings that are treasured by today's world. Nevertheless, the question can be asked, "Was it worth it—not to humankind—but to Gauguin himself?" The nagging feeling that one has deserted one's family combined with loneliness is corrosive to the human spirit. We might not look on Gauguin as a great painter today if he had painted on weekends and holidays. But he might have been relatively self-actualizing and have enjoyed the benefits of a loving relationship and the satisfactions of parenthood.

The wise person realizes that self-actualization is a value. But there are other values.

### Values and Meaning

💡

**Search for the values that are a natural part of human nature.**

Values are to the search for meaning what food is to the hunger drive. Frankl asserts that we have an inborn will to meaning in the same way that we have other inborn impulses. It doesn't seem rational that biology would have given us a hunger drive or a thirst drive if Earth contained no food or water. By the same logic, it doesn't seem rational that nature would have given us a will to meaning if there were no real values to satisfy it.

In the case of human beings, these values are givens associated with the quality of human nature. For centuries we have found it meaningful to be loving to a partner, to raise our children, to provide emotional support to elderly parents, to be genuinely supportive of our friends, to avoid injuring another person, to take care of our health, and to accomplish in accordance with our individual self-actualizing tendencies. These are our basic values. And, really, that's all there is to it. If you fulfill these kinds of values, then your life will have meaning. You *will* avoid the existential vacuum. Doing the right thing, being responsible, will help you feel that life is full, that it makes sense.

### Practice Long-Run Hedonism

🔍

**Realize that living primarily for today's pleasures is a bankrupt approach to life.**

If you live for pleasure alone, particularly today's specific pleasures, your approach to life is called *short-run hedonism*. Short-run hedonism is advocated by one of the world's classical works of literature, *The Rubáiyat of Omar Khayyám*. Khayyám was a twelfth-century poet and astronomer, and his work was made famous in English with Edward FitzGerald's creative translation. The *Rubáiyat* proclaims the importance of pleasure, particularly the pleasure of the moment. One of its famous quatrains proclaims that the author has kicked "barren reason" out of his bed and has taken the "daughter of the vine" (i.e., wine) as a spouse. Another quatrain says that the author would be perpetually happy just to sing in the wilderness with a beloved companion and a jug of wine. Some of the quatrains contain real wisdom, and the *Rubáiyat* is a work of art. Nonetheless, taken as a whole, it preaches a wrongheaded philosophy of life. Living for today's pleasures without an eye on long-run meaning will usually lead to emotional disaster.

Psychotherapist Albert Ellis suggests that we should trade in short-run hedonism for *long-run hedonism*. We should assume that we will live well past today, and that we want to seek some of our payoffs in the future. Yes, we should seek some pleasures in the here and now. But discovering values and finding meaning in life can also be looked on as a sort of pleasure, a psychological pleasure associated with the knowledge that our life has some significance—and this can only be attained by taking a large view of our own life.

### The Reality of Values

**Look upon values as real, not as creations of the human mind.**

Frankl speaks of discovering values. A person who thinks that life is meaningless is like a person in a dark room. There is furniture in the room, but he can't see it. Then he turns on a light, and the furniture is clearly evident. It was there all along. The room was filled with furniture, but it was seemingly nonexistent. Life is like the room and values are like the furniture. The values are there, but the demoralized person may not be aware of their presence. The search for meaning is like turning on the light. Once the light of existential understanding is on, the values appear as solid as furniture—real and apparent. And the existential vacuum, the feeling that life is empty and pointless, vanishes.

Some existential writers suggest that values are creations of the human mind, that they are invented to give our lives the illusion of meaning. It is better to assert that values are real, and that life has actual, not illusory, meaning. If you are dying of hunger in a wilderness, chewing and swallowing a picture of a hamburger and French fries will be of no real use, even if you have the delusion that you are eating food. Similarly, values will fill your life with meaning only if they are discovered and found to actually be there in your psychological world.

And where are these values? How can you discover them? Look back at the strategy that says, "Search for values that are a natural part of human nature." It will help you realize that values are all around you, that your world is rich with potential meaning. You will find that you don't need to look beyond your family, friends, and your vocation in life to find solid values worth living for.

### Choosing to Take a Stand

🔔

**Realize that you can always take a stand against conditions.**

The humanistic viewpoint asserts that you can always take a stand against conditions. This is because you have a free will and can choose your attitude in any given situation.

209

If you accept an attitude of defeat and helplessness, you will tend to suffer a loss of meaning. Your life will be drained of value. If you accept an attitude of success and optimism, you will tend to find meaning restored.

As noted earlier, Frankl points out that even in a concentration camp it was possible to take a stand against conditions. He decided to believe that he would prevail, that he would survive the dangers of the camp, and that he would help others in the camp. The fact that he ultimately did survive is not the point. The fact of the matter is that while he was living in the camp he lived with meaning, not with the despair of an existential vacuum.

Maslow's description of the case of the young woman who worked in a gum factory during the Great Depression also illustrates how it is possible to take a stand against conditions. She returned on a part-time basis to graduate school under adverse conditions, and she restored meaning to her life.

### More Than One Answer

Stop searching for the one meaning in life, but instead discover your set of personal meanings.

More than one person, struggling to make sense out of life, has asked the question: "What is the meaning of life?" However, the question itself poses a problem. It is improperly phrased. It implies that there is such a thing as *the* meaning of life. First, there is no one meaning that is the same for everyone. Frankl notes that asking about the meaning of life is like asking: "What is the best move in chess?" There is no such thing as *the* best move. Best moves depend upon the position of the pieces. Similarly, a meaning in life is distinctive to a given person's situation. If you have to raise one or more children, then a likely meaning of your life is to be a loving and effective parent.

On the other hand, if you have no children, you might find meaning in your vocation or a loving relationship. Or, you might invest your mental and emotional energy in a career that includes a parental role. The novel *Goodbye, Mr. Chips* by James Hilton tells the story of a lonely man who at first is not very well suited to be a teacher in an English school for boys. Then he marries and discovers his nurturing and loving self. His wife dies in childbirth, and the couple's child also dies. Mr. Chips devotes himself to his work. On his deathbed, he overhears two of the other masters talking about him. The first one says to the other, "Poor Chips. Did he ever have any children?" The second one answers, "No. He was married. But his wife died and he was left childless." With great effort Mr. Chips raises himself up a bit, opens his eyes, and looks straight at the two men. "No children? No children, you say? Why I had thousands. And all of them boys." Shortly after, Mr. Chips dies. By deciding to invest his being in his career, Chips was able to find meaning in life, the same kind of meaning associated with parenthood.

There is no reason you can't find value in several life roles. Possibly you will discover meaning in being a parent *and* in loving a partner *and* in the rewards of your vocation. Meaning in life is not limited to a single meaning. I am reminded of a line from the play and film, *Auntie Mame.* Mame says, "Life is a banquet. And most poor fools are starving to death." Life is potentially a banquet rich with an array of meanings.

## *Filling the Vacuum*

🔔

## Watch Frank Capra's *It's a Wonderful Life.*

This movie, familiar to many from its television showings around Christmas, was made in 1946 by director and producer Frank Capra shortly after he returned from duty in World War II. If you're unfamiliar with its still meaningful story, here's a synopsis.

James Stewart plays the part of George Bailey. George is demoralized and thinks his life has no meaning. He contemplates suicide. With the help of his guardian angel, Clarence, George is shown what life in his small hometown would have been like for others had he never lived. His brother would have died in icy water. George rescued him from an ice-skating accident. His mother would be an old, bitter woman with no children. The town's pharmacist would be a self-destructive alcoholic. George stopped him from making a fatal error in a prescription shortly after the pharmacist received the news that his son had died in the war. Many people in the town would have substandard housing because the town's rich old miser would have been able to extract excessive interest from them. (George had headed up a savings and loan association that helped people obtain loans at a reasonable rate.) Finally, George's wife would have ended up an unfulfilled woman without a husband or children. George saw that his life was filled with meaning. It really counted in many ways. He says to Clarence, "I want my life back." And his request is granted. The final scene of the movie shows him a rich man, not in money, but in friends and family. He finally appreciates who he is and what he has.

The important point to realize when watching the movie is that on the outside *nothing has changed*. What has changed is George's perception of life, his psychological world. He sees values where before he saw none. His existential vacuum no longer exists. He loves life and is able to understand with all of his heart and soul that life is, as the title of the film indicates, wonderful.

You will recall Nicholas G., the forty-four-year-old horticulturist who saw life as absurd. As a part of his therapy, he watched *It's a Wonderful Life*. I asked him to take notes on the movie so that we could discuss his reaction to it. Among other comments, Nicholas said, "I see myself as a kind of George Bailey character. I could really identify with what he was going through. And when the film ended I realized that, as George had learned, that my life counted too.

"I asked myself what the life of my wife would be like if I had never been born. She's always told me that I'm her soul mate, the right guy for her. I think she means it. Maybe she wouldn't have had much of a life married to someone else. Who knows? And my two great kids? Well, that's for sure. They wouldn't have been born if I hadn't have been born. How obvious, but how true. What a loss that would have been. And my work as a horticulturist? I lose sight of the pleasure my plants give to people and the way they appreciate my advice.

"I agree with the general notion of the movie that life is what we perceive it to be. Perceiving mine as meaningless, it was. Rethinking some things helps. I'm not sure that I want to say it's a wonderful life. But the thinking I'm doing and watching the movie are helping me see that life does have meaning."

## MASTER STRATEGY 14

*Look upon your neurotic disposition as an asset, not a liability, in your personal search for meaning.*

It is true that by being neurotic you are sensitive to the dangers of an existential vacuum. Being both anxious and aware of the unexpected tricks life can play, you are likely to start thinking about day-to-day existence in negative terms. So it would seem that your neurotic disposition is a liability. But it doesn't have to be this way.

Being neurotic, you almost certainly possess high intelligence, creativity, and a powerful imagination. These are the power tools of your mind. Channel them in the direction of a search for values in your life. You will discover them because *they are there and they are real.*

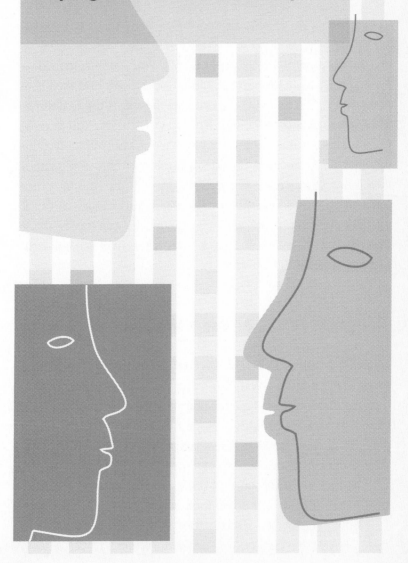

Chapter 15
# Coping with Neurotic Anxiety

**Let's say that** a fire alarm goes off. You are seized with a momentary panic. You are at school or at work and have not been told that there will be a drill. Maybe this is the real thing. Your heart begins to pound. You start to sweat. You experience a sudden muscle tension. You force yourself to find an exit and walk, not run, outside. It turns out there was neither a drill nor a fire. You have just put up with the nuisance of a false alarm. For some reason the system was triggered. But it was not a good reason. Perhaps a prankster was involved. Or there was a short circuit. But, whatever the reason, the alarm did not indicate the presence of an actual fire.

## A False Alarm

Neurotic anxiety can be compared to a false alarm. Something triggers the system—you, the living organism—to respond to a signal that in the end means nothing. The apprehension you experience is groundless. Nonetheless, being neurotic, it seems that you are doomed to experience this sort of thing over and over again.

Walton O., a 6-foot-3 ex-professional wrestler, describes his anxiety this way: "People look at me and think I'm a fearless hulk. The truth of the matter is that I'm a mouse in a tiger's body. I worry about everything. When I drive I always think, 'Today's probably the day I'll get it.' When I go to a movie I keep thinking that maybe there'll be an earthquake and I'll be trapped in the rubble. My blood pressure is high, and the doctor says it's hypertension. There's no physical basis for the problem that he can see. It's probably caused by my constant tendency to worry."

Thelma G., a legal assistant with a secure job and a solid marriage, describes her anxiety this way: "I guess most of us have heard the phrase, 'I'm afraid of my own shadow.' Well, that's me. I think that danger is lurking everywhere. I don't know what to expect. I feel as if something can go wrong any moment—like Chicken Little. If there's a drop of rain, I think the sky is falling. The other day I coughed a couple of times and thought I was catching a cold. I've worked for my present employer, an attorney, for seven years. He's really a sweetheart of a guy, and I know it. Nonetheless, the other day he made a mild criticism of a letter I wrote and I began to think he was going to fire me. I cried when I got home and lost a night's sleep over it. I imagine myself without a job and unable to get one. I overreact to almost everything."

Take note that both Walton and Thelma are describing their anxiety as *chronic*. For them, it tends to be a steady presence over time. They live with it frequently because it is easily triggered. Second, note that they both suffer from *free-floating anxiety*, a kind of anxiety that follows them around like a nebulous cloud. These two attributes are key characteristics of neurotic anxiety. Both Walton and Thelma suffer from *generalized anxiety disorder,* a tendency to worry too much about anything and everything.

What causes a person to suffer from this type of neurotic anxiety? This question was answered in Chapter 3 within the context of the larger question: What causes a person to suffer from a neurosis? In that chapter, we discussed the various viewpoints used to explain the existence of a neurosis in an individual: (1) psychoanalytic, (2) behavioral, (3) biological, (4) cognitive, and (5) existential. I won't repeat the causal factors in neurotic anxiety here. Instead of focusing on *why* you suffer from neurotic anxiety, this chapter will focus on *how* you can reduce anxiety. The self-directed strategies that follow are all designed to help you make life more livable.

## Ways to Reduce Neurotic Anxiety

It is really pretty hard to eliminate neurotic anxiety entirely. Given your neurotic disposition, it is likely that you will have a higher level of anxiety than people who roll merrily along without the slightest notion that something awful can happen to them (or that they might do something awful). People who are irresponsible, arrogant, and unimaginative are often relatively free from neurotic anxiety. They are seemingly born optimists. Your neurosis gives you certain advantages over such people, though. When overconfident people hit a wall in life, they are often incredibly stunned. They have a hard time believing that this could have happened to them. You, on the other hand, are prepared. You have imagined the worst more than once. When adversity does arrive, you are to some extent already desensitized. Now you may find yourself more able to cope than your less neurotic friends.

OK, that's the positive side of neurotic anxiety. However, you still want to reduce its intensity. Why suffer more than you need to? After all, I assume you're not a glutton for punishment. I know that I don't enjoy neurotic anxiety. So I've tried to figure out practical ways to reduce its level in me and in people I have counseled.

Let's roll up our sleeves and do some psychological work.

### The Impulses That You Never Act On

🌱

#### Recognize that you are unlikely to act in an impulsive, irresponsible way.

According to the psychoanalytic viewpoint, much of your anxiety stems from a fear that you will give behavioral expression either to your forbidden sexual wishes or to your forbidden aggressive impulses. These impulses arise from the id, the primitive self. Oh, the impulses are probably there, all right. But they are probably well contained by your inner moral watchdog, your superego. Further restraint comes from your reality-oriented ego.

The fact of the matter is that neurotic people worry a lot about what they imagine they might do, but they seldom do what they worry about doing. On the other hand, people with a psychopathic streak *don't* worry about what they might do. They go ahead and act in an irresponsible way and then have to pay the price for their life blunders. No, you're not that kind of person. You're very cautious. Yes, you worry a lot. But you probably don't get into a heck of a lot of trouble.

Colby L. is a thin, nervous man with a wife two times his size. He makes his living as a clothing buyer for a department store. He says, "In my job I travel quite a bit. I meet attractive women. I've had my share of opportunities. I've had a lot of fantasies. More than once I've thought that I was going to do something that would make me feel terribly guilty the next day. But I've been faithful to my wife for twelve years.

I remember seeing a movie called *The Seven Year Itch*. The married husband in the movie had a chance to go to bed with Marilyn Monroe while his wife was away on vacation. But for all of his desire and her sex appeal, he remained true to this wife. I'm like that guy. It's finally dawned on me that I'm not going to do anything that my conscience won't let me do. And I've got a pretty damned strict conscience. So I'm worrying less about what I might do than I used to. When it comes to sex with other women, I'm a dreamer, not a doer."

You can reduce some of the anxiety arising from forbidden wishes by gaining greater insight into the unconscious level of your mind. Instructions for making a self-analysis were provided in Chapter 12.

## Desensitizing Yourself

❦

### Use the desensitization method to reduce anxiety

Psychologists agree that much of our anxiety is acquired by learning. Basic associations reside behind many of our irrational fears. If a child was locked in a dark closet as a form of punishment, as an adult the individual will likely be claustrophobic, afraid of being trapped and closed in. If a child was bitten by a dog, as an adult the individual will likely have a fear of dogs. Trina H. was subjected to a series of ear operations when she was a preschooler. Today the adult Trina is afraid of doctors.

In a series of experiments supervised by John B. Watson, the father of behaviorism, and his assistant Rosalie Raynor, a toddler known as "Little Albert" was presented with a white rat. Initially, he had no fear of the rat. Then a loud gong was sounded behind him whenever he saw the rat. Quickly, he developed a conditioned fear of the rat. Then it was demonstrated that he also had a fear of a white rabbit, a Santa Claus mask, and a balled-up white terrycloth dishtowel. This second group of fears represents *generalization,* a tendency to respond fearfully to stimuli that are similar to the original conditioned stimulus (the white rat).

In the case of conditioned fears, fears acquired by association, the desensitization method can be very helpful. It is used extensively in psychotherapy, but it can also be self-applied. In order to use the desensitization method, it is not necessary to be consciously aware of the original experience or set of experiences that have given you your phobia. It is only necessary to be aware of the stimuli (i.e., small rooms, dogs, etc.) that trigger your anxiety.

Leila R. was afraid of small bugs such as spiders and crickets in her house. Once she came home at 10 P.M., saw a cricket on the kitchen floor, and immediately went back out her back door. She drove over an hour to stay overnight at a relative's house. Applying the desensitization method, she had a teenage male next door capture a cricket and put it in a bottle. Then the bottle with the cricket was placed on a shelf in her garage. Every day she tried to approach the bottle. The bottle soon contained a dead cricket, but Leila found that, because of generalization, she had a fear not only of live crickets, but of dead ones as well. Each day over a two-week period she was able to come closer and closer to the bottle. The day came when she was able to touch the bottle. In time she could pick up the bottle and shake it. Later, she found that she was able to sweep up crickets and cope with other insects. The method described is called *in vivo* desensitization, meaning desensitization in life. An actual stimulus, such as the captured cricket, is used when this method is applied.

It is also possible to use the desensitization method with self-guided fantasies. Orlando L., a thirty-three-year-old mystery novelist, had a fear of driving a car. He had never taken driver education nor applied for a learner's permit. Using self-guided fantasies, he started with a weak fantasy at first, one not calculated to induce much anxiety. He imagined himself in a car, behind the wheel. He started the motor and sat with the car in the Park position with the motor running. When this fantasy no longer induced anxiety, he increased the anxiety-arousing level of the fantasy. He imagined himself going back and forth slowly in the driveway of his home. Eventually, Orlando was able to imagine himself driving, without anxiety, on a freeway. At this point he had the confidence to take a driver's training course for adults. (Note that at this point the desensitization method switches from self-guided fantasies to in vivo desensitization.)

Today Orlando owns his own car and drives it with a relatively high level of self-confidence.

Orlando drives defensively. He is cautious, does not exceed the speed limit, and is very safety conscious. These behaviors exist because his anxiety level is certainly higher than the average driver's. In this case his anxiety is functional, and it is a good example of how a neurosis can often have unexpected benefits.

### Genetic Fatalism

### Reject the idea that you were born to be neurotic.

The biological viewpoint assumes that neuroticism is an inborn trait. It is further assumed that chronic anxiety arises from this same inborn trait. Consequently, it is to some extent your genetic constitution that gives you your neurotic disposition. There is good evidence that this is true. However, this is true *only to a certain extent.* How much of your neurosis is inborn and how much is acquired is hard to figure out in a given case. Even if your genes are involved, they play only a partial role in your thought and behavior; they're not the whole story. Also, genes influence behavior, but they do not absolutely determine it. That is why you need to reject a genetic fatalism.

You can say, "Poor me. I'm doomed to a life of anxious suffering because of my sensitive, inborn neurotic disposition."

Or, you can say to yourself, "Perhaps I've got an inborn neurotic disposition. But by learning and using various self-directed strategies, I can *modify* the expression of that disposition. I can reduce chronic anxiety by my own thoughtful efforts. I am, within reason, in control of my own emotional destiny."

The second position is the hopeful, optimistic one that you need to adopt as you voyage through live. Refuse to be a patsy to the biological viewpoint. Don't be victimized by the idea that your personality is rigidly created by your genes.

### Avoiding Mistakes in Your Thinking

🔖

### Become aware of your cognitive errors.

Cognitive errors are tendencies to make certain persistent mistakes in the way you think. Two very common cognitive errors are *either-or thinking* and *overgeneralization.* Both errors are capable of intensifying anxiety.

If you are prone to either-or thinking, you tend to see life in all-or-nothing terms. Everything that happens is a Success or a Failure, a Happy Ending or a Tragedy, Happiness or Misery. There is no in between, no shades of gray, no such thing as, "The outcome was so-so." Stanwyck O. is a college student. He is on the honor roll and seeks an A in every class he takes. To him, a B on an exam might as well be an F. When a paper is returned with a B, he thinks, "What a disaster. This is hopeless. Maybe I should drop out of this class." No wonder he suffers from excessive anxiety when he takes an examination. He is falling prey to either-or thinking.

Incidentally, the normal reaction to a B is, "Hey, I got a B! Pretty good. I'm doing all right."

Kimberly H. is going through a divorce initiated by her husband, Davin. She thinks of the future in either-or terms. Marriage stands for happiness and success. Divorce stands for misery and failure. She can see no life for herself after the divorce. She imagines only emptiness and a totally bleak existence. No wonder she is excessively anxious and believes that her life is completely out of control. She thinks, "Without Davin, life is nothing. I won't be able to go on. I don't know what I'll do or where I'll go. Without his love, life holds no pleasure at all."

Kimberly needs to reflect on the way she is thinking. She needs to see that she is making a cognitive error. It is important that she say to herself, "As unpleasant as this process is, as rejected as I feel, there *is* life after divorce. As unlikely as it seems now, I'll meet another man someday whom I can love and who will love me. I know it sounds trite and overworked, but it's really true that when one door closes another one opens. I need to hang on to ideas like that." These kinds of positive, realistic thoughts undercut the adverse influence of the either-or way of thinking. And they will help Kimberly feel somewhat less anxious about her future.

When you overgeneralize, you tend to take one fact and use it to make a general conclusion. The classical example of overgeneralization is Chicken Little, who said that the sky was falling because a drop of rain fell on her head. Schuyler D. is an auto insurance underwriter. An overworked, underpaid worker with a large insurance company, his desk is one of forty similar desks. If his supervisor criticizes an underwriting decision, Schuyler immediately thinks, "I'm going to get fired. Then how will I support my wife and children? Jobs are next to impossible to get these days. I don't know what I'm going to do." He imagines himself homeless and standing in a bread line. In fact he is a valued employee with twelve years of service and seniority. If Schuyler's car motor makes an unfamiliar noise, he thinks, "The motor's probably going to quit on me and I'll be stranded on the freeway." If there is heavy rain for a day, he thinks, "Maybe we'll have a flood and my house will be ruined."

Almost any negative fact can be blown up into a general conclusion. If overgeneralization is one of your cognitive errors, it is a good idea to say to yourself, "I'm overgeneralizing. I don't want to be like Chicken Little. I need to reflect carefully and realize that I'm jumping unnecessarily, and without sufficient basis, to the wrong conclusion."

### Excessive Existential Anxiety

🔑

#### Learn to cope effectively with existential anxiety

As you will recall from Chapter 13, existential anxiety is the fear of death and disability. In and of itself, existential anxiety is not abnormal. It is impossible for a human being to shake such anxiety completely. However, if this kind of anxiety becomes excessive, it interacts with neurotic anxiety and inflates it to an intolerable degree. Turn back to Chapter 13 and apply the coping skills identified in that chapter in your general effort to reduce neurotic anxiety.

### Just Relax

🔮

#### Learn to induce the relaxation response.

The *relaxation response* is a natural response, available to any human being who takes the time and trouble to learn how to induce it. As formulated about twenty-five years ago by Herbert Benson, the relaxation response is an innate pattern that works against anxiety. When you are anxious, you are on high alert. Your muscles are tense; your rate of breathing is rapid. You are in a state of alarm. You are ready to get into a tussle or run away. This is known as the *fight-or-flight reaction*. The relaxation response is antagonistic to this reaction.

It is relatively easy to induce the relaxation response. As with all things, practice helps. So if you keep at it, you will get better and better at inducing it. The response, with self-directed training, becomes conditioned. A kind of psychological pathway develops.

Here are some basic steps that will help you induce the response.

1. Set aside some quiet time when you can be alone and undisturbed for at least fifteen minutes.
2. Sit in a comfortable chair, one that gives you good support and allows your muscles to go relatively limp.

226

3. Close your eyes.

4. Breathe normally.

5. As you breathe in, think, "Re-." As you breathe out, think, "-lax." Each cycle or respiration obviously completes the word *relax.*

6. The word *relax* is a focus word. If you like, you can select another word or phrase that you associate with peace of mind and relaxation.

7. If your mind drifts, don't get irritated. Just go gently back to the focus word. Think of your mind like a child who skips off a park pathway to chase a butterfly or to look at a flower. Without anger, the adult guides the child back to the pathway. Similarly, use your adult self to guide your child self back to the main relaxation pathway.

8. Keep up the relaxation process for about ten or fifteen minutes.

9. Open your eyes when you feel sufficiently relaxed and refreshed.

Research shows that learning to induce the relaxation response can reduce excessive anxiety and may even help some people lower high blood pressure. If possible, you should employ the relaxation response at least three times a week.

### Negative Practice

**Use negative practice to help you cope with obsessive-compulsive behavior.**

One of the most persistent, difficult-to-deal-with syndromes associated with chronic anxiety is obsessive-compulsive behavior. An obsessive idea induces anxiety. Then the anxiety is reduced by a magical ritual. Although the person realizes the ritual is irrational, it becomes an entrenched habit because it has been reinforced a number of times with the positive result of anxiety reduction.

Stephen G. got into his car one morning and immediately had the thought, "I'll probably get killed on the way to work." He decided that if he tapped the steering wheel with both hands seven times that he would arrive safely. The first day he performed the ritual he felt an immediate relief of tension. He arrived safely, and this confirmed the value of the ritual. It seemed to have a positive consequence. The next day he tried to resist the compulsion but ended up tapping the steering wheel. Again, he arrived safely. Although he thought that the ritual was nonsense, he didn't want to take a chance. And the ritual became entrenched.

You will recall that negative practice was defined in Chapter 7 in the context of breaking bad habits. Negative practice consists of voluntarily performing the very behavior that the individual is resisting. It works because the deliberate performance of a bad habit tends to bring it under voluntary control.

Think of the compulsive behavior, the magical ritual, used to reduce anxiety arising from an obsession as a bad habit. In this case, the use of negative practice can be amazingly effective. Stephen was instructed not to resist his tapping compulsion. Instead, he was given the instruction that after tapping seven times, he should voluntarily tap *seven more times* even if he didn't want to. He didn't want to. It seemed really silly. But he did as instructed. After about ten days, he gave up the compulsion completely. An involuntary behavior was brought successfully under voluntary control.

Instead of fighting compulsions, negative practice allows you to use a sort of psychological jujitsu on them. You undermine them by going with, instead of against, their energy. You can apply negative practice to help you manage almost any obsessive-compulsive behavior pattern you may have. (Refer back to Chapter 7 for a more complete exposition of the nature of negative practice.)

---

**MASTER STRATEGY 15**

### Work to make a distinction between imaginary threats and real ones.

When you feel anxiety, ask yourself, "What is the source?" If the source of anxiety is objective and real, if there is a well-defined threat to life and limb or to your self-esteem, then you're entitled to be anxious. To be free of anxiety when there is real danger is as abnormal as to experience anxiety when there is no danger at all. In fact, the proper word when there is real danger is *fear,* not anxiety.

How can you distinguish a real threat from an imaginary one? Ask yourself, "Am I using either-or thinking? Am I overgeneralizing?" Let your common sense be your guide. Your rational, reality-oriented mind will give you the right answer in most instances. Once you decide that your imagination is working overtime, say to yourself, "This is neurotic anxiety, not real fear. And I refuse to be intimidated by a fantasy." Consciously and deliberately thinking along these lines will do much to dampen useless anxiety.

# Chapter 16
# Coping with Neurotic Depression

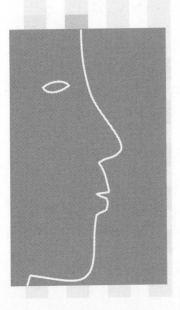

**Depression.** Winston Churchill, the prime minister of England during World War II, called depression his "black dog." Like an unwanted mongrel, it followed him around for many years, nagging and barking at him, making his life miserable.

The excessive consumption of brandy, cigars, and rich food was one of the self-destructive ways Churchill coped with depression. Painting pictures, political activity, and writing books were three of the constructive ways that this outstanding leader coped with depression. He never rid himself entirely of his depressive tendencies, but he learned to manage them and to minimize their effects on his life.

Depression has no respect for fame or fortune. It strikes the rich and the poor without discrimination. Some writers have compared it to an emotional plague. It has been known as a scourge of humankind since ancient times. The father of Western medicine, the Greek physician Hippocrates, referred to depression as *melancholia*. He believed that it was caused by the bodily humor (i.e., fluid) black bile. Note that *mela-* is a combining form meaning "black."

Estimates suggest that about 10 percent or 20 million people in the United States suffer from mild to severe depression. No wonder depression is often called the common cold of mental illness. If it is persistent and nagging, like Churchill's "black dog," it is chronic depression, and that is the kind of depression that we're concerned with here.

## Signs and Symptoms of Depression

If you are in fact depressed, you probably already know it. It is quite common for someone to remark, "I'm depressed." Nonetheless, depression is a sometimes confusing syndrome consisting of a set of signs and symptoms. So here's an informal checklist that will help you describe and define your own depression, if you suffer from it.

1. *A low mood.* This is the principal symptom of depression. Depressed people are often conscious of having the blues or the "blahs." Alana C., a full-time homemaker with four children, says, "I am conscious of whole weeks that seem to me like I'm living in a dull, gray world without color or charm."

2. *Lack of pleasure in life.* Nothing seems like fun anymore. The joy seems to be gone from existence. Everything is boring. Even sex brings little satisfaction.

3. *Sleep disturbances.* Either you suffer from insomnia or you sleep too much. Moderately depressed people often find it difficult to get a full night's sleep. On the other hand, severely depressed people often sleep ten hours a day or more.

4. *Eating disturbances.* Moderately depressed people tend to overeat or indulge in binges. However, severely depressed people tend to lose appetite and often become too thin.

5. *Walking and talking slowly.* Bodily actions slow down. Everything seems to take too long to do. Even a simple task such as washing dishes feels like a next-to-impossible burden. It is as if you have weights attached to your arms and legs.

6. *Chronic fatigue.* This symptom is obviously closely related to the behavior identified in number 5. You feel tired all of the time. Chronic fatigue associated with depression can

easily be confused with *chronic fatigue syndrome,* a medical condition involving residual viral effects and an autoimmune reaction. The chronic fatigue linked to depression is primarily psychological in nature.

7. *Thoughts of suicide.* Moderately depressed people do not seriously entertain killing themselves. They're still in there trying to fight and cope with life. Severely depressed people often take the idea of suicide more and more seriously. If you fall into this category, it is essential that you seek professional help as soon as possible.

## The Four Faces of Depression

The basic portrait of depression has already been sketched. However, depression has more than one face. Clinical psychology and psychiatry recognize four basic kinds of depression: (1) dysthymia, (2) cyclothymia, (3) major depressive disorder, and (4) bipolar disorder.

### Dysthymia

*Dysthymia* is synonymous with what I have been referring to as moderate depression. The depression is chronic, often spanning months and years. Dysthymia is the same thing as neurotic depression. It is depression arising from internal biological or emotional sources, not from the objective facts of your life. In other words, human beings can sometimes be depressed when, in a sense, there's nothing much to be depressed about. The word *dysthymia* is from Greek roots. *Dys-* means "bad" or "difficult," and *thymia* refers to mood. Thus the literal meaning of the term is essentially "bad mood."

### Cyclothymia

*Cyclothymia* is a mood that cycles, that changes from "bad" to "good" to "bad" again. The bad mood is moderate depression. The good mood is *hypomania,* meaning a mania that is below psychotic proportions. The individual is *not* out of touch with reality and often functions well during periods of hypomania. Stanley E., a television screenwriter, often takes on two or three contracts for scripts at a time. He bites off almost more than he can chew, but not quite. When he meets his obligations, receives his checks, and can theoretically enjoy himself, he has to endure an emotional crash. He falls into a depression that lasts until the cycle repeats itself. Cyclothymia, like dysthymia, is essentially a version of neurotic depression.

### Major Depressive Disorder

*Major depressive disorder* is characterized by severe depression. Even if the depression has only existed for a few weeks, a psychiatrist may be able to diagnose it as a major depressive disorder. This is because there are suicidal thoughts and often a risk of real suicide. This disorder does not yield readily to self-help strategies, and anyone suffering from it should seek professional assistance.

### Bipolar Disorder

*Bipolar disorder* is characterized by the negative pole of depression alternating with the positive pole of mania. During the manic phase, thinking is so irrational that the individual is out of touch with reality. Linette W., an insurance agent, believed during a manic phase that she could win the Miss America contest, invent a new kind of tanning lotion, and drive across the country all within a two-week period! She was in a state of excitement and agitation for about a week. Then everything seemed to collapse around her and she fell into a major depressive phase. Bipolar disorder, like major depressive disorder, requires professional treatment.

## Why Are You Depressed?

There is no single cause of depression. Instead, there is a set of causal factors that interact to create depression.

First, there are *psychosocial stressors*, events that trigger depressive episodes. You lose a loved one, get divorced, go broke, and so forth. No wonder you're depressed! But depression based solely on such negative events is not neurotic. There would be something wrong with you if you were not at least temporarily depressed.

However, psychosocial stressors can be magnified in importance. Some people may perceive a cutting remark made by a friend, a bad grade on an examination, a failure to be promoted, and similar events as catastrophes. When such stressors trigger depression, then the depression can be thought of as neurotic in nature.

Second, there are *biochemical factors*. Hypoglycemia, or low blood sugar, can induce a depressive state. Low levels of certain chemical messengers in the brain, particularly serotonin and norepinephrine, are associated with depression.

Third, depression can be influenced by *psychodynamic factors*. In psychoanalysis, the self is seen as a field of conflicting forces. A common interpretation of depression is that it represents repressed rage. Lisa F. believes that her husband dominates her and completely controls her life. However, she is a traditional woman who is convinced that she must love and respect her husband. Also, he intimidates her with his aggressive personality. So she seldom speaks up and she bottles her feelings. At a psychological level, this translates into depression.

Fourth, *learned helplessness* can be an important factor in depression. A personal history of failure in a particular arena of life, or a set of bad experiences, may cause you to overgeneralize. You will tend to think that you're helpless in situations in which you are not actually helpless.

There are other causal factors, and some of them will emerge as we explore what you can do for yourself in your efforts to manage depression.


## Ways to Cope

How should you react to depression? The following set of self-directed psychological strategies offer you effective ways to cope with neurotic depression. Employing them will minimize the adverse impact of depression on your life.


### *Watching Your Diet*

❡

#### Significantly limit the refined carbohydrates in your diet.

As already noted, low blood sugar can play a role in depression. The excessive consumption of refined carbohydrates will induce *hypoglycemia,* or low blood sugar. This is

237

because of a phenomenon known as the hypoglycemic rebound. When blood sugar is elevated too quickly, the pancreas overreacts and secretes too much insulin. This causes a rebound effect, and the blood sugar plunges to a below-normal level.

What are refined carbohydrates? Everyday table sugar is a principal source. You will find it in soft drinks, baked goods, ice cream, and most desserts. Also white flour and white rice are quickly digested and act much like sugar. The same is true of some nonprocessed foods such as potatoes and some varieties of rice. Every food has a *glycemic index,* a measure of the rate at which it converts into blood sugar. There are books that publish such index tables, and it is a good idea to become familiar with such information.

In addition, the excessive consumption of refined carbohydrates tends to deplete your body of B-complex vitamins. This is because these vitamins play an essential role in the conversion of sucrose and other carbohydrates into glucose. However, the B-complex vitamins are also essential in the process by which neurons synthesize chemical messengers. So if your levels of B-complex vitamins are low, then your levels of serotonin and norepinephrine are also likely to be low. Low levels of these chemical messengers are believed to be principal culprits in depression.

### Keeping Things in Perspective

🔎

### Resist mental magnification.

*Mental magnification* is a tendency to enlarge the psychological size of the undesirable things that happen to you.

As noted earlier, you might be giving psychosocial stressors, adverse events in your life, too much attention and value. Recognize that mental magnification is a neurotic tendency.

Robert A. has one-half of his life savings invested in municipal bonds. They tend to be relatively stable securities. Nonetheless, he used to study the market report every day. He says, "If a bond dropped a couple of points, I would think, 'Oh, no, I'm going to lose everything. I'll probably go broke before I know it.' I would be down in the dumps all day. Now I've trained myself to think, 'So Bond A went down a couple of points. It's no big deal.' Bonds have to bob up and down a little, like corks in an ocean. The important thing is that the bulk of my capital is untouched and my payments from the bonds are fixed."

Whatever happens to you, try to put it into perspective. Take the long view. Avoid pumping up a minor event into a major one.

### Becoming Assertive

❦

**Work to acquire assertiveness skills.**

I mentioned earlier that one psychodynamic interpretation of depression is that its core consists of repressed rage. Depressed people often feel used and abused by others. One of the principal reasons they feel this way is that they give other people too much power. A spouse, a best friend, a parent, a supervisor are often granted, without much resistance, a dominating role. They, on the other hand, take on a passive role. This automatically encourages the other person to become more aggressive. They, in turn, become more miserable.

It doesn't have to be this way. If you've given others too much power, you can turn things around. You can take back what you have given away by using assertiveness skills. *Assertiveness* is a way of interacting with others that is neither passive nor aggressive. It is the happy middle ground between the two.

Following are some important assertiveness skills. Both clinical experience and research in psychotherapy have shown that neurotic people can often put these skills to work in their lives.

1. *Use I-messages, not you-messages.* An I-message states how you feel. It *does not* label the other person's actions. Say, "I feel hurt," not, "You're always putting me down." Say, "I'm full," not, "You're pushing food on me." Say, "I'm not going to do it," instead of, "Stop always telling me what to do." You-messages tend to be aggressive. Not wanting to be aggressive, and not thinking in terms of an I-message, you may often fall silent and allow yourself to be controlled. The I-message gives you a powerful alternative.

2. *Speak with feeling and conviction.* This is an assertiveness skill known as *feeling talk.* Listen to the voices of passive, overly agreeable people. You will find that they tend to sound flat and spiritless. You have to speak up, be heard, and have a moderate amount of emotional content in your speech. This does not mean your voice has to take on an aggressive, hostile tone. Listen to the voice of a news anchor you admire—male or female—and note how the anchor's voice has a warm, convincing quality. Model your own speech patterns after the role model.

3. *Repeat requests more than once if necessary.* We have all heard the saying, "If at first you don't succeed, try, try again." The same thing goes for making requests. This assertiveness

skill is called *broken record*. You can use it to get a partner to do something he or she resists doing. You can use it to return defective merchandise. Sometimes people say, "If I have to get my way by using broken record, then I don't want my way. I want the other person to *want* to do what I want him or her to do." Maybe this is asking too much. You want cooperation at a behavioral level. Don't seek compliance at a deeper level. If you don't agree with the philosophy of broken record, all right. But be prepared *not* to get your way in many life situations.

Assertiveness skills will help you short-circuit the frustration and associated depression that arise from ineffectively dealing with other people.

### Taking Responsibility

🔦

**Reject the idea that you are genetically fated to be depressed.**

You should reject the idea of genetic fatalism. This same advice was given in the context of neurotic anxiety (see Chapter 15). It is repeated here particularly because modern psychiatry tends to place much of the blame for depression on genetic heritage. Research does suggest that genes play a role in depression, particularly in the cases of major depressive disorder and bipolar disorder. Nonetheless, genes don't tell the whole story. You are a conscious individual with the ability to think, reflect, and take voluntary action. As this chapter and other chapters have revealed, there is much you can do for yourself. The self-directed strategies in this chapter will show you how you can work around your depressive tendencies and greatly minimize their impact on your daily life.

Steven G., a professional tennis player, says, "I used to blame my genes for being depressed. My father suffered from depression. But I've come to see that assigning all of my blue moods to my genes is just another rationalization, a way of not taking responsibility for my behavior."

### Avoiding Cognitive Errors

🔍

#### Take a hard look at the way you are thinking.

As explained in the last chapter, cognitive errors can induce or aggravate anxiety. The same is true of depression. The two errors of either-or thinking and overgeneralization often play a role in dragging you down into emotional quicksand.

Kyra T., a part-time piano teacher, says, "If I got a C on a test I would think, 'I failed the test.' If my husband criticized me, I would think, 'He doesn't love me anymore.' If my child was disobedient, I would think, 'I'm completely blowing it as a mother.' Either-or thinking was my nemesis. And it was pulling me down into the emotional dumps for no good reason. I've tried to purge either-or thinking from my mental life and, as a consequence, my emotional life is much better."

Harrison O., a certified public accountant, says, "If any little thing went wrong I would think, 'There it goes again. Murphy's Law. It applies to me. If anything can go wrong, it will. It always happens to me. Something always goes wrong.' Now I think, 'Nothing *always* goes wrong. That's ridiculous, an overgeneralization. Sure, some things go wrong some of the time. And some things go right some of the time. It's an obvious lesson to learn, but I've been a little slow in learning it. Now that I have, I can verify that I have less problems with depression than I used to."

### Going Easy on Yourself

💡

#### Don't be too self-critical.

Neurotic people tend to have an overactive superego. Their inner police officer is forever catching them in minor errors and transgressions and turning them into major crimes.

Washburn L. made an arithmetical error and overpaid a phone bill by $100. When the company caught the error and gave him a credit on his next bill, he felt stupid. He told himself, "I'm an idiot. I can't be trusted with paying the bills. I'm really a blockhead."

Sylvia L. put herself on a 1,200-calorie-per-day diet. She stuck to it like glue for ten days. Then she had a 700-calorie hot fudge sundae on top of her regular food for the day. She told herself, "You're hopeless. You have no willpower. You'll never lose weight."

Washburn needs to tell himself, "Anyone can make a mistake once in a while. To err is human." Sylvia needs to tell herself, "I'm not perfect. Who is? So I broke out of diet prison. It's a natural reaction. When I do, I've got to take it in stride and calmly return to my eating program."

The habit of being too self-critical is a significant factor in depression. But you don't have to let your superego rule your mental roost. You can interrupt the process by thinking, "I'm not going to let my superego ruin my life. It's just an inner police officer gone berserk. I'm a nicer, better, more competent person than it tells me I am."

### *Moving Beyond Past Failures*

🔆

### Don't let learned helplessness get you down.

A substantial body of research has shown that learned helplessness plays a significant role in depression. Learned helplessness is acquired by a series of adverse experiences. Warren G. was bad at math in grammar school. He had no aptitude for it. Now as an adult when he has to balance his checkbook or compute the interest on a loan, he blocks. He thinks, "I'm no good at math. I can't do this."

Jasmine E. was married for five years to a charismatic, controlling attorney. He was able to win every argument they had and often made her feel like a fool. In her second marriage, when she and her husband begin to have a misunderstanding, Jasmine fails to be assertive. She thinks, "I can't win. I never do. He'll just make mush out me if I try to explain why I think I'm right about this." So she clams up and suffers in silence.

Both Warren and Jasmine need to realize that they are making a transfer of feeling from earlier situations to present ones. Warren can say to himself, "I'm an adult now, not the helpless child I was in grammar school. Maybe Warren-the-adult has capacities that Warren-the-child did not have."

Jasmine can say to herself, "My first husband made his living with his verbal fluency. I really was pretty helpless when I dealt with him. But my second husband, although normal in intelligence, is no whiz kid with his mouth. Maybe Jasmine-in-her-second marriage isn't nearly as helpless as Jasmine-in-her-first-marriage."

Learning to tell the difference between actual and learned helplessness will assist you in coping with depression.

Here are some ways to recognize the presence of learned helplessness:

- You have a history of repeated failure experiences in an important life arena such as work, school, child rearing, or marriage.
- You tend to treat a new situation as if it is an older, similar situation.
- You often feel that you just can't cope with the challenges of life.
- You know that you are bright and able, but you feel incompetent and ineffective.
- You find yourself threatened by, and even avoiding, what could very well be opportunities.
- You have a severe case of "giveupitis"—you give up before you have made a sustained effort to succeed.

### Getting Stuck in a Role

Refuse to derive benefit from the role of Depressed Person.

There is a difference between being a depressed person and the social role of Depressed Person. Being depressed is an actual mental and emotional condition, as already outlined and discussed. Playing the role of Depressed Person is a way of extracting payoffs from being depressed. You can get out of household chores and even going to work. Lana S. says, "Whenever I got depressed, my husband became Mr. Nice Guy. I never got so much attention. I had to talk long and hard to myself not to fall into a pattern of self-indulgence. The real depression brought the benefits. The benefits made me play the role of Depressed Person to the hilt. My husband, poor guy, what could he do? He saw my depression as something beyond my control, and he was only trying to help. It was up to me to see the difference between being really depressed and playing a part. When my actual depression began to lift, I made it a point to pick up my responsibilities one by one. And it helped my mental health."

## MASTER STRATEGY 16

### Act as if you are not depressed, and it will help your depression lift.

William James, as mentioned before, once said that his first act of free will was to believe in his own free will. And this helped his own depression lift because he saw himself not as a passive victim, but as an agent of his own destiny. So, like James, reaffirm a belief in your own free will.

James, along with a physiologist named Carl Lange, formulated a well-known theory of emotions known as the *James-Lange theory*. This theory states that actions can induce feelings. Applying the theory to depression, the argument runs that if you act as if you are not depressed, it will help your depression lift. "But how can I do this?" you protest. "I'm depressed!" This is where free will comes in. The theory does *not* say you can will away your depression. To feel depressed is an involuntary response. However, you can will your actions. You can move and behave in a way that is not a good fit with depression. You can bathe, wear clean clothes, be well groomed, smile at others, and say pleasant things.

The positive feedback you receive within yourself and from others by acting as if you were not depressed will help the actual depression lift.

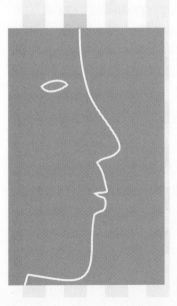

**Chapter 17**
# Coping with Neurotic Anger

**Think of Old Scrooge,** the miser. The central character in Charles Dickens's short novel *A Christmas Carol,* Scrooge is a perpetual grouch. He criticizes his nephew, an employee, for little or nothing. He can't see why people are happy during the Christmas season, and declares "Bah, humbug!" when he sees holiday activity. He is an angry man—and for no good reason. He has a lot to be thankful for. His kind of anger— chronic and without meaningful purpose—is the subject of this chapter. It is neurotic anger.

Granted, Scrooge is a fictional character. But I'm confident that Dickens based him on some people he knew. The perpetual grouch is a type. Hippocrates recognized such individuals as having a *choleric* personality trait. He believed that their bodies produced too much yellow bile. To this day, when someone gets angry, we sometimes say that his or her bile is rising. Well, we're not going to approach anger in terms of bile. It's an antiquated and incorrect theory. Even though Hippocrates was incorrect about the physiology of anger, he was still a good observer of human behavior. So let's agree that this world has more than its fair share of Scrooges, grouches, choleric personalities—call them what you will.

Angry people make others suffer.

But they also suffer themselves. If you are a chronically angry person, this chapter will help you manage this destructive emotion and lessen its impact on your life and the lives of others.

## Signs and Symptoms of Neurotic Anger

What is neurotic anger?

It is an unjustified, excessive, and aggressive response to the frustration associated with another person or situation. It can be acute or chronic. When it is acute, it can be a transient flare-up, like the burst of flame that quickly comes and goes on a match. When anger is chronic, it is like a slowly burning fuse. The two kinds of anger are related. A slowly burning fuse can lead to an emotional bomb and a psychological explosion. Such an explosion, acute in nature, is described with words such as *fury* or *rage*.

The following list of signs and symptoms are associated with neurotic anger, and will help you recognize its presence.

1. *High blood pressure.* About one-half of the people who suffer from high blood pressure do so without a known organic basis. This kind of high blood pressure is called *essential hypertension*. An important causal factor is chronic anger.

2. *Psychosomatic symptoms.* Migraine headaches, ulcers, skin rashes, and backaches are either induced or aggravated by the emotional stress associated with anger.

3. *Verbal hostility.* Angry people often make cutting remarks, listen poorly, interrupt others, and "wittily" produce thinly veiled insults.

4. *Inability to relax.* Chronic anger is associated with muscle tension. When you are angry, it is difficult to just let go and calm down.

5. *Muscle pain.* This is linked to items 2 and 4. We hear a lot about *fibromyalgia,* or chronic muscle pain, these days. In many cases, fibromyalgia has a biological basis. It is possibly an autoimmune disorder somewhat similar to rheumatoid

arthritis. However, the emotional stress associated with neurotic anger is likely to aggravate muscle pain.

6. *Disturbed interpersonal relations.* People who suffer from chronic anger often have fallings out with others, make enemies, have unhappy marriages or get divorced, and are frequently alienated from their children.

7. *Rash, impulsive, ill-considered decisions.* Angry people often "rush in where angels fear to tread." They want things to happen *now,* and they don't want to wait to gather more information or think things through.

## Why Do You Suffer from Neurotic Anger?

Let's assume that you suffer from neurotic anger. Why?

As with most psychological problems, there is no one easy answer. A constellation of interacting causal factors plays a role. Some of these are identified here.

First, as with many behavioral problems, there is evidence to suggest that a tendency to be an angry person is an inborn trait. We may call this trait *hyperaggressiveness.* It is a fairly stable, predictable trait, and it often appears in preschoolers. Studies suggest that when a preschooler is rated as hyperaggressive, the tendency tends to still be present in adolescent and adulthood. Research indicates that about 15 percent of children are "difficult." These are the kids who tend to become angry adults.

Second, some children suffer from *attention deficit disorder,* or ADD. This disorder is often partially outgrown in early adolescence. But it can also carry over to some extent and have an effect on the emotional life of adults. Attention deficit disorder has become one of those "wastebasket" labels that are overapplied. Nonetheless, there is evidence that it is to some extent a real condition. If you suffer from it, it will aggravate your neurotic anger.

Third, as we all know, some people were spoiled as children. Alfred Adler, a pioneer psychotherapist and personality theorist, said that a child tends to become spoiled when the parents (1) do not set well-defined limits on behavior, (2) are overindulgent, (3) give too much easy gratification, (4) make the child feel too special without any real basis, and (5) yield to the child's desires in almost all situations. To Adler, a spoiled child is impulsive, self-absorbed, and quick to anger. The same traits often appear in adults who were spoiled children.

Fourth, angry people are often egocentric. The world revolves around them. They can see only their own point of view. Being self-absorbed, they find it difficult to fully realize that others actually exist as living human beings with real thoughts and feelings. Instead, egocentric adults tend to perceive others more or less as things, mere cardboard figures, to be manipulated and controlled. And, of course, they find their anger rising when others won't dance to their tune.

Fifth, neurotic anger tends to be associated with a lack of self-actualization. People who feel that they are barking up the wrong vocational tree or that they have followed the wrong road in life are likely to feel frustrated. If a person's talents and potentialities are going to waste, then that individual's dissatisfaction with life is often experienced as anger. Agatha G., a life insurance broker, says, "I like the income I make from insurance sales. But it's not *me*, not the real me. I've always wanted to sing and dance and perform. It's what I did best in high school. But I feel that something in my soul is being neglected."

Sixth, a person who suffers from chronic anger may have

an overblown sense of justice and injustice. "Right is right and wrong is wrong!" he or she thunders. If the person is a parent, the slightest breaking of a rule by a child calls for a swift thunderbolt of punishment from Mount Olympus. Huxley O. took his parents, wife, and children out for a Mother's Day brunch at a hotel. When he received the check, a 15 percent gratuity had been added to the bill. Huxley could accept this, but the gratuity had been levied on the sales tax as well as the hotel's charge. Huxley saw red, declared this to be grossly unfair, and approached the manager in an aggressive manner. The manager made an adjustment, but Huxley fussed and fumed for the rest of the day over the fact that they had tried to rip him off.

Seventh, perfectionism and chronic anger often go hand in hand. A perfectionist frequently demands that everything be in order, that the house be spic-and-span in an almost military sense, that a spouse and children behave in exactly the way the perfectionist expects, and so forth. Any deviation from his or her wishes is a basis for a blowup. Perfectionists tend to make the same hard demands on themselves that they make on others. Darlene L. says, "If I don't pay my bills on time, have plenty of clean clothes, have a car with no squeaks or grime, and have my files in logical order at work, I freak out. I get upset and can't settle down until things are just the way I know they should be."

## What You Can Do for Yourself

If you suffer from neurotic anger, there is a lot that you can do for yourself. Following you will find a group of self-directed psychological strategies that will help lower your emotional pressure. You have to live with others, and these strategies will help your human relationships. However, you also have to live with yourself. The art of managing anger will make you more emotionally comfortable. It will make your life much more pleasant.

### Re-examining Your Thinking

💡

#### Challenge your own thought processes.

This same basic suggestion has been made in the context of coping with both neurotic anxiety and neurotic depression. But it bears repeating here. In the same way that the cognitive errors of either-or thinking and overgeneralization can induce anxiety and depression, they can induce anger.

Gail E., a grammar school teacher, mother, and wife, says, "I used to go out to dinner and if even one thing wasn't to my liking I got mad about it. I was angry with the restaurant and the server, but I took it out on my husband and kids. Obviously, I was letting either-or thinking rule my mind. I would think, 'This dinner is a disaster.' And the basis of this thought was simply that the baked potato was dry when the rest of the dinner was excellent. As a result of several sessions with a therapist who emphasizes the re-examination of your own thought processes, I've learned to get rid of a lot of either-or thinking."

Tyler A., a grocery store manager, says, "I was frequently angry at the employees. I would think such thoughts as, 'Why does Susan always stack the shelves wrong?' or, 'Bill never does what I ask him to do when I want to do it,' or, 'Mary never gets to work on time.' Learning to challenge my own thought processes revealed to me that Susan usually stacked the shelves properly. When she did not, that's when I would use the word *always* in my mental processes. The same goes for the word *never* applied to Bill and Mary. I was making behavior that was in reality an exception to ordinary behavior into a kind of general rule about the way these workers act. I had to look long and hard at the way I think to fully appreciate this. And my level of anger has subsided. Sure, I get irritated. But that's reasonable."

### Dealing with Life's Frustrations

🔍

#### Practice time-delay frustration tolerance.

One of the primary sources of frustration is when we have to wait for things to happen. We wait for long red lights to change, we wait for tables when restaurants are crowded, we wait for someone who was supposed to show up at a particular time and place, and so forth. We can't control these delays. And they *are* frustrating. However, persons who suffer from chronic anger have little or no tolerance for them. A delay of even a few minutes can make their blood boil. They rev up their motors when the light is red or honk their horns at drivers in front of them.

They ask a restaurant's host several times, "Is my table ready yet?" A husband shouts at his wife, "You kept me waiting forever!" In fact he was waiting seven minutes.

One way to undercut a tendency to overreact to time delays is to impose them on yourself when you don't actually have to wait. For example, let's say you want to have a snack or, if you smoke, a cigarette. Invert a three-minute egg minder, and tell yourself that you'll wait until the sand runs down before you eat or smoke. If you are away from home, use your wristwatch in the same way. Use short, self-imposed time delays before you make a phone call, go for a break at work, turn on the radio, and so forth. This will automatically build your tolerance for frustration, and you will find that it will tend to transfer in a beneficial way over to situations over which you have no control.

## Taking Your Time

### Slow down when you want to speed up.

That's right. The advice seems paradoxical, but there's something to it. First, one of the characteristics of angry people is that they suffer from what is called sometimes called the *hurry-up sickness*. They are impatient with the rate at which events occur. This was obvious in the descriptions of behavior associated with time-delay frustration. However, the hurry-up sickness also makes them try to act and complete tasks on a double-time basis. They wash and dress at a furious pace, eat breakfast in big bites, speed on the road to work, talk rapidly, write rapidly, and in general are running, running all day.

The hurry-up sickness is associated with the Type A behavior pattern, first identified in the late 1950s by the cardiologists Meyer Friedman and Ray H. Rosenman. Aggressiveness, or chronic anger, and hurrying are linked. When they appear together, as they do in the Type A pattern, then the combination becomes a risk factor in heart disease.

And the sad thing is that all the hurrying up doesn't do much good. You don't get things done much faster when you rush. Let's say that Jim and Tom have to make the same roughly one-hour trip. The route is a combination of freeway and surface-street driving. Jim cuts in an out of traffic, jumps stop signs, tailgates, and sometimes breaks the speed limit. Tom doesn't dawdle, but he doesn't rush either. He drives assertively, not aggressively. And he has an eye on safety. Road engineers have found that, on average, a driver like Jim will arrive at his destination only a few minutes earlier than a driver like Tom will.

Rushing through life is pointless. You are more likely to make mistakes or have accidents. These can make events take *more* time, not less. You've probably heard the saying, "Haste makes waste." Well, it's true.

Learn to make haste slowly.

### The Downside of Multitasking

🔋

### Don't try to do two things at once.

Associated with the Type A behavior pattern is a tendency to want to do two things at once. For example, you are talking to a friend on the phone, get somewhat bored, and decide to write checks for bills while giving half your attention to your friend. Or, you insist on talking on your cell phone while driving. Or, you write a letter to a friend while a teacher is lecturing. All of these behaviors betray a nervous restlessness.

Doing two things at once is a form of self-induced stress. It works against relaxation and contributes to your overall level of anger. It is a form of self-induced time pressure. You are trying to squeeze too many happenings into a limited period. Instead, do your best to give your full attention and interest to one task or subject. You will find that, over all, it contributes to mental and emotional calmness.

### *Taking the Bigger View*

🔋

### Avoid a small, mean view of life.

Angry people tend to look at life in a very limited way. They nitpick. They criticize. They fuss over details. They are like a person walking through a beautiful park who focuses only on details near his or her feet—the cracks in the sidewalk, a few weeds in the grass, the fact that a park bench needs paint, and so forth. The individual misses the rustle of the trees in the light wind, the flight of a flock of birds, the warmth of the shining sun, and similar aspects of a larger experience. As you travel through life, don't focus on the cracks in the sidewalk and the weeds. Take a longer view.

Old Scrooge took a small, mean view of life. And what did it get him? Loneliness, unhappiness, poor digestion, and ghosts in the night!

The only day you can live is *this* day, this set of twenty-four hours. You can look upon this day as a burden filled with obstacles and frustrations. Or, you can take a larger, more expansive view of life and recognize that this day is precious. You have the option to look upon it as a challenge filled with opportunities and rewards.

### *Getting Outside Yourself*

🔋

### Be aware that egocentrism is a prime source of anger.

Egocentrism is a mental trait associated with the thinking of preschoolers. They can see no point of view other than their own. Three-year-old Vito is banging on a set of drums. His mother says, "Please, Vito. Stop! I have a terrible migraine headache. I have to have some peace and quiet so I can relax." Vito stops banging the drums as requested. Then he looks within himself trying to find this mysterious something called a "migraine headache." He can't find it. So his thinking runs along these lines, "If I don't have this thing called a headache, Mom doesn't have it either." So he begins banging his drums again, much to his mother's dismay. Vito is not simply being disobedient. He actually believes that Mom doesn't have a headache if he doesn't have one.

In the view of preschoolers, the world revolves around them. Four-year-old Felicity was traveling with her parents at night when there was a full moon. She kept looking out of the window at the moon. At last she asked her parents, "Why is the moon following us?" They told her that the moon is in its own orbit and isn't following anybody. "Oh, no," said Felicity. "It stops when we do. And it starts when we start. And it speeds up when we do. And it slows down when we do. It's following us." Felicity was a good observer. At a perceptual level, the moon *was* following them.

Egocentrism, natural in the preschooler, is difficult to give up. It is a sign of emotional immaturity when an adult still thinks in egocentric terms. Unfortunately, this is often the case. Roy G., a thirty-four-year-old married man with two children, says, "I used to suffer from a sad case of childish egocentrism. When my wife and I started to discuss something—anything from raising the kids to how to spend some money—I never even made an effort to see her point of view. I just looked at my own way, and my way was, by definition, right. And I would get angrier and angrier with her. Seeing as my way was, as far as I was concerned, the only way, I felt enormously frustrated with her. I thought she was a blockhead. In reality, I was the blockhead. Marriage therapy, and a technique the therapist used called 'reverse role playing' has taught me that my wife can think and understand as well as I can. She has a point of view that is valid in its own way. I don't have to always agree with it. But at least I make an effort to see her point of view. It has done a lot to help me diminish the steady-state anger that was undermining the quality of my life and my relationship with my wife."

Tell yourself, "Egocentrism is for preschoolers. I'm not a preschooler. I'm an intelligent adult who can see a point of view other than my own."

### Controlling a Need for Power

Get off your power trip.

People who suffer from a high level of neurotic anger are often on a power trip. The informal phrase *on a power trip* suggests an individual who has a high need for power. This psychological need is well recognized in a standardized psychological test known as the Thematic Apperception Test. The test consists of a set of cards that portray persons in various situations. The drawings are deliberately ambiguous, allowing them to be interpreted in different ways by different individuals. The test is called a *projective test,* because it is based on the assumption that what you say about the cards are projections from your subconscious mind. One of the principal aims of the cards, when used in clinical settings as a diagnostic tool, is to reveal an individual's set of more or less stable motives. One of these motives is the need for power.

A subject taking the test is instructed to tell a short story about each card. The story is to have a beginning, middle, and end. Also, the subject is supposed to say what at least one person in the card is thinking and feeling. Kay G. looks at a card portraying a male and a female walking among grass and trees. The male is carrying a basket. Kay says, "This is an engaged couple going on a picnic. He wants to stop under the first tree he sees. But she insists that they keep going until they can eat by the lake. They enjoy the lunch that she has fixed. He doesn't like roasted chicken, but that what she's made. He would rather have cold cuts, but she says that if he's going to be her husband, she doesn't want him dying of a heart attack from eating too much fat. So she's setting him straight right from the very beginning. Later, they go boating even though he wanted to loaf and take a nap. She's thinking that this is a fine day and is feeling good about life."

Kay's projection identifies her clearly with the female in the card. Her story is transparent, and her need for power is blatant. The day must go her way. She needs to dominate and be in control. It is easy to see how in real life a person like Kay is bound to suffer from quite a bit of anger. In real life, unlike the fantasy world, it is not possible to always dominate and have absolute control. People who try to be little dictators in human relationships are bound to become emotionally upset. Other human beings are not puppets and they will not always dance to the strings you pull.

It is important to realize that a lot of anger is generated by a high need for power. If you have such a need, look for ways to bring it down to a more normal level. Tell yourself, "The excessive need for power, like egocentrism, is a sign of emotional immaturity. I would like to have my way, but I can't always get it. I'm going to back off and get off my power trip. I don't need to be the boss every time in every situation."

### Choosing a Different Fate

🌡

### Once again, reject a genetic fatalism.

As in the case of anxiety and depression, it is important to reject a genetic fatalism in association with anger. It is true that, as mentioned before, the tendency to be an angry person may be a carryover from an inborn tendency to be hyperaggressive as a child. However, you are *not* doomed by genetic messages. You must, of course, cope with what they dictate. And this is the purpose of the self-directed strategies described in this chapter. Your intelligence, your capacity to think, gives you freedom of choice. Chronic anger does not need to be your fate.

### Dealing with Attention Deficit Disorder

🌡

### Look for ways to counteract the possible effects of attention deficit disorder.

I don't want to say that all people who suffer from chronic anger also suffer from an adult version of attention deficit disorder. But in some cases it can be a complicating factor. If you think that this is so in your case, there are several basic things you can do to neutralize the effects of this disorder. Fortunately, these interventions are mild and prudent.

First, restrict the sugar in your diet. This suggestion is somewhat controversial from a medical viewpoint. Some researchers say that sugar has no effect on attention deficit disorder and hyperactivity. Others insist that too much sugar elevates blood levels, making you temporarily "hyper" and then depressed. As excessive sugar can do you no good, it's probably better to be safe than sorry. So cut down on refined sugar when and where you can.

Second, avoid foods with artificial flavors and additives. This is a basic suggestion made by many pediatricians to the parents of ADD children. The same tip goes for you. Foods in boxes and cans often are highly modified. Within reason, and as much as possible, buy fresh fruits and vegetables. Buy unprocessed meats. Drink water and milk, not soft drinks.

Third, you should be aware of the beneficial effects that coffee can have on attention deficit disorder. Children with ADD often take prescription stimulants. These often have a paradoxical effect on the condition, tranquilizing ADD children instead of stimulating them. The same is true for coffee with these children, and this beverage should be tried before prescription drugs. Coffee contains caffeine, a powerful cerebral stimulant. (Tea also contains caffeine.) So if you think that an adult form of ADD is aggravating your emotional life, give coffee a chance.

### *Realizing Your Goals*

**Don't neglect your need for self-actualization.**

As indicated earlier, a lack of self-actualization can be frustrating and it can intensify your general sense of anger toward life. This is not the first time in this book that I have referred to the need for self-actualization. You need to become the person you were meant to be. For your emotional health, you need to pursue goals that reflect the real you, your real talents and potentialities. However, as I have also said, you don't have to put all of your eggs in the self-actualization basket. Don't destroy the rewarding aspects of your life in the name of self-actualization. You can be self-actualizing on a part-time basis.

Agatha G., the life insurance broker who was quoted earlier, says, "I'm sticking with life insurance sales as a job. But now I'm taking singing lessons and performing in local productions of musicals. I just got a part in *Fiddler on the Roof*, and I'm thrilled."

### Why So Serious?

🔦

**When you feel your anger rising, say to yourself,
"Life is too serious to take it seriously."**

There is a big difference between life *being* a serious matter and *taking* it seriously. When you take life too seriously, you intensify your emotions. Irritation becomes anger. Everything is magnified. Everything is given excessive importance. It is because life itself is so important, because you don't want to suffer from the physical and emotional suffering that anger can induce, that it is to your great advantage to focus on the larger picture—life itself—instead of its minor, passing events.

## MASTER STRATEGY 17

### Recognize that neurotic anger is self-induced, manufactured by your thoughts and perceptions.

Your mind creates neurotic anger. And your mind can dissolve it. The various strategies presented in this chapter, if applied to your emotional life with a positive attitude, can help you manage your frustrations and aggressive tendencies in constructive ways.

Can you rid yourself of all your anger? No, of course not. If you have something to be really angry about, then anger can sometimes be an appropriate reaction. But this is seldom the case. A neurotic disposition may make you hot under the collar when the appropriate reaction might be mild irritation. Emotional maturity requires that responses such as anger or irritation be correctly matched to the events that trigger them.

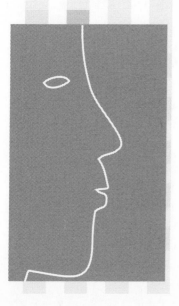

# Chapter 18
# Getting Along Without Pills

**If at all possible,** you should cope with your neurotic symptoms without pills.

Why?

First, psychiatric drugs are not a cure for mental and emotional problems. They are *treatments*. They may help you manage a problem. In this sense they can be useful, but they certainly are not panaceas. Don't expect to find peace of mind and the key to living in a bottle.

Second, all psychiatric drugs have potentially adverse side effects, which range from mild to severe. Many side effects are very distressing. Before you take a drug, prescription or otherwise, look up its side effects. Almost all drugs are listed on the Internet, and it is easy to find out quite a bit about them. You can look them up by their generic name or their capitalized trade name.

Third, it is possible to become overly dependent on drugs. Instead of taking responsibility for your behavior, you may lose much of your motivation to grow as a person. You expect the drug to do the fixing. The drug, which in most cases is not really fixing anything, provides the false promise of a psychological world free of dark clouds.

Make no mistake about it. You want to get along without pills if you can. (I am, as you probably realize, using the word *pills* loosely to include any psychiatric drug, whether administered by pill, tablet, capsule, or syringe.)

I am well aware that psychiatric drugs are useful and even necessary in the treatment of some conditions. This will not be a muckraking chapter that says all pill taking is, by definition, bad. However, I do take the position that ingesting pills for what ails you at an emotional level should be a last resort not a first choice.

## The Varieties of Psychotherapy

The literal meaning of the word *psychotherapy* is a healing of the self. This is accomplished without drugs. That is why psychotherapy, when first pioneered by Freud with the method known as psychoanalysis, was nicknamed the "talking cure." Psychotherapy uses skills and techniques that rely heavily on language and the kind of comprehension that accompanies our understanding of words.

Because I believe you should make an effort to use non-drug approaches before you start taking pills, brief descriptions of the various kinds of psychotherapy follow.

1. *Psychoanalysis* tries to help you develop insights. It stresses the importance of self-understanding and is based on the ancient dictum, "Know thyself." Or, as the philosopher Socrates put it, "The unexamined life is not worth living."

2. *Behavioral therapy* is based on principles of learning. It assumes that many of your emotional problems are, in a sense, bad habits. It helps you find ways to break or modify these habits.

3. *Cognitive therapy* helps you think more clearly and realistically. It assumes that cognitive errors induce adverse emotional reactions such as anxiety, depression, and anger.

4. *Humanistic therapy* is designed to assist you in exploring your need for self-actualization. Also, humanistic therapy supports your search for meaning in life. It helps you take a hard look at your existence and the way you live in your unique psychological world.

5. *Existential therapy* is a term some authors and professionals use instead of humanistic therapy. There is little difference between the two terms. If a difference can be assigned, humanistic therapy emphasizes the positive, optimistic side of self-exploration. Existential therapy emphasizes overcoming demoralization and despair.

6. *Hypnotherapy* takes advantage of the fact that human beings are often highly suggestible. Neurotic conditions are often induced by autosuggestions, the things we tell ourselves with our self-talk. These self-defeating autosuggestions can often be countered with positive suggestions offered by a hypnotist.

Although Freud often used hypnosis in his early work, he gave it up in favor of the techniques he pioneered in association with psychoanalysis. But there are still quite a few professionals who see a place for hypnotic suggestion within the framework of psychotherapy.

7. *Multimodal therapy* combines the best elements of the kinds of therapy that have already been described. Most contemporary psychotherapists see merit in all approaches and draw the best from them. In most cases if you seek psychotherapy, you will not encounter a therapist who insists on one and only one way of doing things.

If you do seek psychotherapy, remember that you need to *participate* in your recovery. Recovery is a process requiring your active cooperation. You can't just sit back and expect a therapist to repair or fix you. It's not like taking a car to a mechanic. If you do decide to seek psychotherapy, reading and applying the principles presented in this book will facilitate the process.

## Kinds of Psychiatric Drugs

It is a good idea to know something about the basic kinds of psychiatric drugs. They are so widely prescribed that it is important to know what you can expect from them. In the following section, I briefly describe the various kinds of drugs used to treat mental and emotional problems. Every drug has a generic name (uncapitalized) and a trade name (capitalized). There are many drugs within each group I've identified. In each case, there is at least one example of a drug with both its generic and trade name.

1. *Antipsychotic drugs* are also called the "major tranquilizers." These are used to treat psychotic symptoms, symptoms often associated with schizophrenia. Schizophrenia is a serious mental disorder characterized by delusions, or false ideas. These delusions are often accompanied by hallucinations, which are false perceptions involving vision, hearing, or other senses. One of the principal ways that antipsychotic drugs work is by regulating the activity of dopamine, a chemical messenger in the brain. The drug clozapine is often marketed under the trade name Clozaril. The drug chlorpromazine is often marketed under the trade name Thorazine.

2. *Antidepressant drugs* are used to treat various kinds of depression. In general, these drugs work by regulating the activity of chemical messengers in the brain. Two messengers,

or neurotransmitters, of particular importance are norepineph-rine and serotonin. When prescribing these drugs, the physi-cian assumes that the patient has low levels of these neurotransmitters. The drug phenelzine is often marketed under the trade name Nardil. The drug fluoxetine is often mar-keted under the trade name Prozac.

3. Lithium carbonate is used to treat bipolar disorder. As a consequence, it is called a *mood-stabilizing agent* because it modulates the extremes of mania and depression. The action of lithium carbonate is not too well understood. However, it appears to work by promoting optimal activity among some of the brain's chemical messengers. A natural mineral salt, lithium car-bonate is often marketed under the trade name Lithotabs.

4. *Stimulants* are used to treat attention deficit disorder (ADD). As I mentioned earlier, this condition can occur in adults as well as in children. When a person has a genuine case of ADD associated with a dysfunction of central nervous system arousal, a stimulant can have a paradoxical, and consequently beneficial, effect on the process of attention. The drug methylphenidate is often marketed under the trade name Ritalin.

5. *Antianxiety agents* are also called the "minor tranquil-izers." They are used principally to treat the chronic anxiety, and some of the other symptoms, associated with neurosis. These drugs work by lowering central nervous system arousal; excessive alertness decreases to some extent. They also tend to induce a certain amount of muscle relaxation. Lowered arousal and relaxation are incompatible with anxiety, so when they are induced, anxiety tends to diminish. The drug diazepam is often marketed under the trade name Valium. The drug alprazolam is often marketed under the trade name Xanax.

If you are neurotic, it is highly unlikely that you will receive a prescription for an *antipsychotic drug*. However, under certain circumstances any of the other drugs mentioned might be prescribed. In practice, you will be most likely to receive a prescription for either an antidepressant drug or an antianxiety drug.

## Living Without Psychiatric Drugs

The aim of this chapter is to help you find a way, if at all possible, to live without psychiatric drugs. In fact all of the self-directed psychological strategies offered in prior chapters are drug-free in nature. They involve looking at yourself from a psychological standpoint, an approach that emphasizes not your biochemistry but your mental and emotional life as a functioning human being. The following self-directed strategies, with the exception of the first one, are based on the assumption that you are not presently taking a psychiatric drug. Their goal is to help you avoid becoming enmeshed in a closed circle of drug taking from which it is often difficult to escape.

### *Changing Gradually and Safely*

🔔

#### Don't quit a psychiatric drug cold turkey.

If you are presently taking a psychiatric drug, and you have a strong motivation to live without the drug, don't quit cold turkey. Some people, fed up with the idea of being dependent on a drug or unhappy with side effects, stop abruptly. This can have serious negative consequences. There can be a boomerang effect, and your symptoms may become temporarily worse. Or there can be withdrawal symptoms that are so unpleasant they may send you running back to the drug for relief.

It is important that you give up a drug gradually. To do this, you need the help of a physician or a psychiatrist who understands drugs and who can offer you at least some supportive counseling or psychotherapy.

### Considering Other Options First

**Make pills a last resort for your emotional problems.**

These days when people have psychological or emotional problems, they often automatically think in terms of medication. Psychiatric drugs are frequently the first treatment of choice. I encourage you to place them *last* on your list of options.

The order of your efforts to cope with the symptoms of your neurosis should proceed as follows:

First, take advantage of the self-directed strategies presented in this book. Do all you can to help yourself. If you are neurotic, you are also almost certainly intelligent and creative. Turn these attributes toward the all-important task of self-rescue. Think of yourself as your own therapist. After all, who knows you better than you do?

It is sometimes said that the person who acts as his or own attorney has a fool for a client. I have heard the same logic applied to therapy and self-improvement. But I don't agree with it. You *can* be the agent of your own mental health. In the same way that you may have dug an emotional hole with your thoughts and your attitudes, you can find psychological stepping stones and toeholds that will bring you up to level ground. No matter how low you are or how helpless you feel, start today to look upon yourself as your prime resource.

More than one person, on his or her own, has found the inner strength to cope with neurotic symptoms. And, remember, none of the self-directed strategies offered in this book involve the taking of drugs.

Second, if you can't seem to be sufficiently effective on your own, seek the assistance of a qualified psychotherapist. The principal professionals who offer psychotherapy alone, and who do not prescribe drugs, are clinical psychologists. Clinical psychologists hold Ph.D. degrees and have usually had substantial training in all modalities of psychotherapy.

If you seek psychotherapy, remember that you need to participate in your recovery. Recovery is a process, and it requires your active cooperation. You can't just sit back and expect to be repaired by a therapist. Even if you do decide to seek psychotherapy, reading and applying the principles in this book will facilitate therapy.

Third, if psychotherapy is ineffective, you can turn to psychiatry. Psychiatrists hold medical degrees and can prescribe drugs. They are also qualified to offer psychotherapy. Although any physician can prescribe psychiatric drugs, I encourage you to consult with a psychiatrist, a specialist in mental and emotional problems, before you actually start taking a drug.

### *Managing Not Curing*

**Recognize that pills don't cure.**

It is unfortunate, but true, that many people who seek drug therapy expect the pill to cure their mental and emotional problems. The pills don't cure. Anybody who knows anything about the subject recognizes this. The pills help you manage your problem. They play a role similar to that of insulin therapy in the treatment of diabetes. Taking prescribed insulin helps the individual manage his or her illness. But a cure is not expected. Also, note that the condition is managed better if the patient understands the illness, eats correctly, controls his or her weight, and exercises moderately. Similarly, even if a psychiatric drug is used, self-directed psychological strategies can play an important role in the successful management of emotional problems.

It is important to do what you can for yourself, even if you take a pill. If you have unrealistic expectations about what a pill can do, if you expect miracles, you are likely to be disappointed.

### Maintaining Proper Brain Chemistry

**Increase levels of the brain's chemical messengers with prudent eating habits.**

Low levels of norepinephrine and serotonin are associated with depression. Levels can be increased with antidepressant drugs. However, levels can also be increased with prudent eating habits.

This territory was covered earlier. Nonetheless, for review and emphasis, let's note once again that sugar and refined carbohydrates tend to deplete the body of B-complex vitamins. These same vitamins are involved in the synthesis of the brain's chemical messengers. Consequently, a diet that is rich in natural nutrients and scant in refined carbohydrates will help you fight depression.

274

Also, it is a good idea to take a multivitamin capsule on a regular basis. Be sure that the formula contains plenty of B-complex vitamins. Although a vitamin capsule is a pill, it is not a psychiatric drug.

If at all possible, it is better to fight off biochemical depression with smart eating than with psychiatric drugs.

### Encouraging Natural Chemicals

Boost your endorphin levels with moderate exercise.

Endorphins, like norepinephrine and serotonin, are chemical messengers found in the central nervous system. The word *endorphin* is a contraction of the two words *endogenous* and *morphine*. In other words, endorphins are natural morphine-like substances. Unlike drugs that are ingested, endorphins are generally thought of as beneficial. They help us fight pain and enhance our sense of well-being, and they definitely help us fight depression. It is a good idea to boost your endorphin levels.

It has been found that moderate exercise can accomplish the result you are looking for. And what is moderate exercise? Take a brisk twenty-minute walk three times a week and you have exercised moderately. That's all there is to it. Perhaps you prefer to jog, run, swim, or ride a bicycle. Whatever your preference, the exercise should be sustained and aerobic.

## Understanding the Psychological Effects of Drugs

### Recognize that drugs have a placebo effect.

The placebo effect is the capacity of a pill or almost any treatment to mobilize your positive expectations and turn them into results. (The word *placebo* is derived from Latin, and means, "I shall please.") The placebo effect is powerful. In an experiment subjects who are given a placebo, a pill without any active ingredients, often report improvement. A headache feels better. Or, arthritic joints don't seem as stiff.

The placebo effect is not limited to physical ailments. It also applies to psychological distress. When you receive a treatment for your mental and emotional problems, you will almost always feel better at first. The treatment can range from taking a drug to psychotherapy. Anxiety is reduced. Depression lifts. Then, often, the symptoms return. The honeymoon is over. The spell cast by the placebo effect dissipates because the effect is only temporary. It works at the beginning of a treatment, but it is hard to sustain. After the placebo effect wears off, the treatment is really effective or it is not. It must stand on its own merits.

A wise old physician, quoting generations of other old wise physicians, once said, "You've got to take a new drug while it's still curing." The remark is, of course, cynical. If the drug has real value, it keeps on curing. If the drug is worthless and derives its temporary benefit from the placebo effect, it will stop curing. Of course, it never "cured" in the first place. Although cynical, the remark is also based on a realistic appraisal of the facts. Many "cures" have existed in the history of medicine. For example, during the nineteenth century,

London physicians prescribed the ground-up hair of the bear in honey for bald men because the bear is a hairy animal. It is easy to imagine a young man, desperate to keep his hair, looking in the mirror and telling himself that the hair-of-the-bear treatment seems to be working. Only after a period of time has passed without real, sustained results will a worthless treatment be discontinued.

All treatments, including psychotherapy, carry a placebo effect. This is true not only of worthless treatments but also of those that actually work. You need to recognize that the placebo effect is temporary. After it is gone, the treatment stands on its own. This recognition will help you deal with the frustration and disappointment you are likely to experience when you begin to realize that a treatment is not working miracles. It can help, but it can't work the wonders that are often projected upon it by wishful thinking.

In the event that you do decide to take psychiatric drugs or seek psychotherapy, approach either treatment with a realistic attitude. Expect good results, but don't expect magic. If there is a placebo effect, which is likely, it will wear off. Then you will have to work intelligently with the treatment and the professional who administers it to obtain sustained beneficial results.

### Abusing Food and Alcohol

🍄

**Don't self-medicate with alcohol and food.**

If you avoid prescription drugs for your emotional problems, there is still the risk that you will turn to two other very common nonprescription "drugs." These are alcohol and food. It is widely recognized that alcohol is a drug. But food is not usually thought of as a drug. I am using the word *drug* very loosely here. Food has the capacity to dull the senses and, like alcohol, lower central nervous system arousal. Eating triggers the parasympathetic activity of the nervous system. Consequently, it acts as a natural tranquilizer. If you eat a lot or binge, the effect on the body and the mind is much like taking a prescription antianxiety agent. The same is true about alcohol.

The abuse of both alcohol and food is common because both provide temporary relief from emotional distress. Recognizing this fact, you need to look for long-term relief from your personal problems. Employing the self-directed strategies in this book will help you reach this goal and will simultaneously help you avoid the trap of either alcohol abuse or food abuse.

Here are some ways to identify patterns of alcohol and food abuse in your own behavior:

- You eat or drink to tranquilize yourself.
- You eat or drink when you feel sorry for yourself.
- You eat or drink when you are bored.
- You eat or drink when you are angry. This can include either anger that you blame on others or anger directed toward yourself.
- You tend to think of food in exaggerated terms such as "fantastic," "incredibly delicious," "delightful," and so forth.
- You drink in order to nurture a creative process such as writing or composing music.

## MASTER STRATEGY 18

### *Challenge the idea that you need psychiatric drugs.*

You should be sure to make a distinction between a *need* and a *desire*. People often confuse the two. A person will say, "I need a new refrigerator." What the person really means is, "I want a new refrigerator because the one I have now, although perfectly functional, doesn't have an ice maker and doesn't match the colors in kitchen since I repainted it." The new refrigerator is not needed; it is merely desired.

In a similar way, if you are suffering from chronic anxiety or depression, you want relief. You may think that you need a pill because a drug holds forth the promise of quick relief without significant effort on your part. I have tried to show you that this is often not true. Even if the drug does offer some promise of relief, similar results can be obtained in many cases with self-directed strategies and/or psy-chotherapy. Granted, you have to put more personal effort into the recovery process. But the evidence available from research on psychotherapy suggests that the results will often be as good as those achieved by taking drugs. And the results are more stable and sustained because you have made a personal investment in them.

If you suffer from schizophrenia or from bipolar disorder, then it is likely that you require drug therapy to get any relief. However, this book is not addressed to people who suffer from those conditions. It is addressed to neurotic people. Assuming that you are one of these people, I grant that you have emotional liabilities. However, research also suggests that you probably have substantial strengths that will help you offset these liabilities. As I have mentioned before, two of these strengths tend to be intelligence and creativity. You can harness these strengths as two mental workhorses that will pull you out of the quicksand of your emotional life.

*(continued)*

### MASTER STRATEGY 18

## Challenge the idea that you need psychiatric drugs.
### (continued)

The odds are very high that you are what psychotherapists informally refer to as "a good, healthy neurotic." If so, although you have problems, you also generally function well, are responsible, and have more power available for the self-management of your problems than you sometimes give yourself credit for.

Give yourself and your mental faculties a chance before you decide that you need pills.

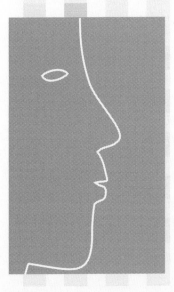

# Chapter 19

# Squeezing Lemons into Life's Lemonade

**If you are neurotic,** you probably think that life hasn't handed you just one lemon, but a whole bag of them.

You say to yourself, "Why me? Why do I have to have hang-ups? Why was I picked out by some malevolent fate to suffer? I wish I were happy and well-adjusted like other people."

Beryl G., a forty-two-year-old architect and a single mother of two children, said in her first psychotherapy session, "I don't know why I have to be loaded down with a neurosis. It's like a bad dress that I can't give away and that some damned fool forces me to wear every day. I want to be strong and noble and courageous like the architect Howard Roark in Ayn Rand's novel *The Fountainhead*. He was a person who lived for his ideas, not to please others. I, instead, am weak and wishy-washy and let myself get pushed around. I worry about everything. I get depressed if I think a client doesn't like my ideas. And I bend myself into a pretzel to please. I bring no integrity to my vocation."

Perry A., a thirty-eight-year-old married high school teacher with four children, said in his first psychotherapy session, "I go around thinking that other people are smarter than me, better looking, and more competent. I wish I were more like this person one day and more like that person another day. I'm too short, an ineffective father, a hopeless lover, and a muddled teacher."

In this chapter, I'll try to show you that the kind of negative appraisals made by Beryl and Perry are not only useless, they are based on false assumptions. There is no reason to feel sorry for yourself if you, like them, have a neurosis. On the contrary. Let's explore why you have a lot to be thankful for.

## Inferiority Complexes

A person can have not only one, but several, inferiority complexes. The same individual may have an *I-can't-do-math* inferiority complex, an *I'm-not-pretty* complex, and an *I'm-too-short* complex. Another person might have an *I-can't-tell-a-joke* complex, a *nobody-likes-me* complex, an *I'm-too-fat* complex, and an *I'm-not-a-good-athlete* complex.

Where do inferiority complexes come from? According to Alfred Adler, the psychologist who coined the term, an inferiority complex arises because the will to power is frustrated. German philosopher Friedrich Nietzsche first proposed the concept of the *will to power*. He said that we have an inborn desire to become effective and competent. If this desire, the will to power, is frustrated, as it often is, we tend to develop one or several inferiority complexes, depending on what goal or aim we are unable to achieve. When I was in the fifth grade, I wanted to be able to do arithmetic problems as well as the other kids. I couldn't. So I developed an *I-can't-do-math* complex. When I was in high school, I wanted to be a normal weight and attractive to females like the other guys. Instead, I was about 50 pounds overweight. So I developed an *I'm-too-fat* complex.

Your set of inferiority complexes is your bag of lemons.

## *The Principle of Compensation*

Alfred Adler said, "The human being has a great capacity to turn a minus into a plus." Or, to put it another way, it is possible to squeeze a lemon and make lemonade.

I remember the first time I drank actual lemonade. I was a child of seven, and I drank a glass on the porch of a couple who owned a chicken ranch in San Fernando, California. The lemonade was cold, sweet, and delicious. Then I tasted a lemon directly from one of their trees. The lemon was warm and sour. I couldn't believe that the lemonade came from lemons. But I soon learned that the secret of the magical transformation was the way in which the lemon juice had been combined with sugar and cold water.

Your sugar and water for turning lemons into lemonade are your intelligence and the principle of compensation.

You don't have to be the perpetual victim of your inferiority complexes. You can transform them into assets. For many years, Charles Atlas ran advertisements proclaiming that he had been a 98-pound weakling. He successfully operated a mail-order course advocating a system for gaining greater strength called "dynamic tension." Atlas actually had been a 98-pound weakling at the age of sixteen. And as a mature adult he won prizes for his excellent physique. He also made a lot of money from his correspondence course. Fitness expert Jack LaLanne provides a similar example. He had been an asthmatic child, and transformed himself into a man of great strength. Both Atlas and LaLanne put the principle of compensation to work in their lives.

The twentieth-century author Aldous Huxley had vision in only one eye. And in that eye, he had tunnel vision. It is as if he had to read everything through a tube held up to his eye.

He became one of the best-read persons in the literary world of his day. He also wrote such admired books as *Brave New World* and *Point Counter Point.* He used compensation to prove that his handicap was only an impediment to his talent, not an absolute obstacle. (Alfred Adler was an ophthalmologist before he became a psychologist. He obtained many of his ideas about the process of compensation from observing the behavior and attitudes of his eye patients.)

## Success Through Compensation

I have already mentioned that I had a mathematics inferiority complex. One of the reasons I became a psychologist is that I was using compensation to offset my lack of arithmetical skill. When I was younger, I used word fluency and verbal comprehension as my counterweights on the scale of academic ability. I figured that I could go far as a psychologist even if I couldn't crunch numbers. Much to my dismay, I learned in my third year of college that a course in statistics is required to obtain a B.A. degree in psychology.

I thought I was sunk. I believed I couldn't do it. But there was no way out except to try. I decided to give the statistics course twice as much study time as any other individual course. I worked many problems on scratch paper. I passed the course with a C, and I felt I was fortunate to obtain a grade that was good enough to meet graduation requirements. I also learned that I could do math if I compensated with a lot of extra effort.

Again, much to my chagrin, I was required to take more statistics in graduate school for a master's and a doctorate. Well, I had to bite the bullet. So again I applied myself. In the end I actually took an advanced statistics examination in place of one of two foreign language requirements for the Ph.D. (Statistics is, in a sense, a "foreign" language.) And I have taught introductory statistics at the college level a number of times. All in all, the principle of compensation when applied to my math complex served me well.

One of the reasons I majored in psychology was that I wanted to use psychological principles to help me lose weight. By the age of twenty, I had decided that my compulsive eating was due to a neurosis. I thought that I could compensate for that neurosis by gaining insight into my own personality and by applying habit-breaking principles. It worked. I lost 70 pounds over a period of two years. A number of years later, when I had earned a doctorate, I worked as a therapist with overweight clients. My experiences culminated in the book *Think Yourself Thin: How Psychology Can Help You Lose Weight.* The paperback version of the book went through twenty printings. Again, the principle of compensation was operating. I turned the minus of my adolescent obesity into the plus of helping others and writing a successful book.

Think about this for a moment. If I had not been bad at math as a child, I would have not become a psychologist. I might have become a physicist or an astronomer. Those fields attracted me, but I avoided them because I thought I didn't have the mathematical ability they required. Today I'm very grateful that I instead became a psychologist. I appreciate the understanding that it has given me of myself and of others.

Also, if I had not been obese as an adolescent, I would not have written my first book, *Think Yourself Thin.* This book helped me launch a highly rewarding part-time career as a nonfiction author. So, in a way, the negative factors in my early life were—odd as it sounds—gifts. They were my lemons. And I needed them to make my own particular kind of lemonade.

The Italian actor-writer-director Roberto Benigni won the 1998 Best Actor Academy Award for his role in the film *Life Is Beautiful*. Accepting the award, he said, "I want to thank my father for the gift of poverty." What he meant was that if he had not experienced poverty as a child, he would not have had the understanding and sensitivity required to identify with persons who are deprived and underdogs. If he had not been a poor child, there is no way he could have achieved what he accomplished as a writer and actor. He compensated for his early deprivation, and it brought him to the heights of professional achievement.

## What You Can Do for Yourself

Think of your hang-ups as challenges that have a great positive potential. They are not permanent obstacles on the road of life. A rewarding, effective life is not denied to you because of your neurotic tendencies. On the contrary, you can, through the principle of compensation, often convert liabilities into assets. It is possible to do a lot for yourself. In the following sections I present a group of self-directed psychological strategies that will help you squeeze your personal lemons into lemonade.

### What Complexes Really Are

Recognize that an inferiority complex is
just a set of ideas you have about yourself.

An inferiority complex is just that—a *complex*. A complex is a set of interrelated ideas you have about yourself. It is not necessarily "true" in any objective sense of the word. However, if you believe that the complex is true, then it becomes a self-fulfilling prophecy. You act as if it is true and it becomes, for you, the truth. So you need to say to yourself, "My inferiority complex very likely consists of a set of ideas I have acquired through unfortunate experiences. This set of ideas may be wrong. I have an inferiority complex, but that doesn't mean I'm actually inferior."

As I mentioned, I had a math inferiority complex as a child and an adolescent. Why? Was I really inferior in my mathematical aptitude? Maybe. But looking back I doubt it. I went to several grammar schools and was often placed in a class that was doing work I was unfamiliar with. So, missing important information, I had a hard time catching up and understanding what was going on. As a child I didn't see this as a failing in the educational process but as a failing within myself. I developed ideas such as "I can't understand fractions" or "I can't move a decimal point correctly" or "I can't understand long division." This set of "I can'ts" became mental obstacles, obstacles that were very difficult to overcome. But they were in fact imaginary figments of my childish imagination.

All inferiority complexes are similar. Kiki S. has an appearance inferiority complex. She thinks that both her nose and her mouth are too big. She believes that she is tall and gawky with tiny breasts. She says, "I look at myself in my mirror and I can't believe that any man would be attracted to me. I remind myself of a crane, one of those ugly long-necked, long-legged birds." The odd fact is that Kiki makes her living as a fashion model. Most men think of her as stunning. Kiki is a lovely woman. But she doesn't perceive herself that way.

Kiki's negative self-image is related to the way she was treated as a young child by classmates, older siblings, and her mother. Taller than average for her age, and thin, she was given various nicknames such as "Wire Hanger," "Flagpole," and "Alien." Nicknames are almost always negative, and they affect self-perception. Also, Kiki's mother had an authoritarian personality. She was very critical of Kiki and sometimes called her an "Ugly Duckling."

Kiki's inferiority complex can't be overcome with plastic surgery. Her face and body are fine. She needs a change in inner perception, one that helps her recognize that her inferiority complex has no more reality than she assigns to it.

Here are some ways to recognize the presence of an inferiority complex in yourself:

- You tend to see yourself as actually inferior, not usually recognizing that this is an *idea* about yourself that may not be objectively true.
- You tend to think that other people are more intelligent, better looking, or more competent than you are.
- You have a history of being made to feel inferior when you were a child—either by peers, siblings, or your parents.
- You worry a lot about being liked or accepted by others. You care too much what other people think of you.
- Even when you have a significant success or achieve an important goal, you still have a nagging sense of inadequacy or incompetence.
- You feel anxious and nervous in many social situations because you doubt your ability to relate effectively to others.

## *A Positive Life Position*

🎈

### Reject the "I'm not OK—you're OK" life position.

The concept of a life position is part and parcel of the theory of transactional analysis. *Transactional analysis* is a behavioral theory that helps us better understand the ways in which we interact with other people. The father of transactional analysis was the psychiatrist Eric Berne, and his way of thinking gained fame with the general public when his book *Games People Play* became a bestseller about forty years ago.

The "I'm not OK—you're OK" life position is associated with inferiority complexes and low self-esteem. If you adopt this position, you tend to see yourself in negative terms and other people in positive terms. You are too short or too tall. Everybody else in the world has a just-right stature. You are too skinny or too fat. Everybody else in the world is a normal weight. You are not very intelligent. Everybody else is brilliant. You are not clever. Everybody else is a genius. Well, you get the idea. You have a distorted perception of yourself because you use others as a yardstick for judging yourself, and you come up lacking. In fact you also have a distorted perception of others because you tend to think that they have more on the ball than you do. And, in fact, they're people just like you. And they have their own problems and flaws.

Don't take a backseat to anybody. You're just as good as they are. And, with all their flaws, other people are OK too. This is the healthy life position. In transactional analysis it's called the "I'm OK—you're OK" position.

And how do you move from a self-defeating position to a life-enhancing position? You *decide*. Yes, that's it. It's your decision, your choice. According to Berne, you have an Adult ego state, a rational, thinking self that can make good decisions. You also have a Child ego state, an impulsive, emotional self that is likely to make bad decisions. It is your Child ego state that puts you in the "I'm not OK—you're OK" position. Being aware of both ego states, you can voluntarily say to yourself, "I'm going to make important decisions from my Adult ego state, not my Child ego state. One of my first important decisions will be to decide that I am rejecting the 'I'm not OK—you're OK' position and that I am accepting the 'I'm OK—you're OK' position."

Beryl G., the architect, and Perry A., the high school teacher, introduced in the first pages of this chapter, learned to reject the "I'm not OK—you're OK" position. After several sessions of psychotherapy, Beryl said, "I regret ever comparing myself to Howard Roark and thinking of him as an ideal type. I recognize that he was arrogant and selfish and egocentric. I'm none of those things. He wouldn't do anything to please a client. I will. That's my nature. I like to satisfy other people when I can. And there's nothing wrong with that. Instead of thinking of myself as wishy-washy, I'm beginning to think of myself as a person who can negotiate intelligent compromises."

Toward the end of the therapy process, Perry said, "If I think clearly, and I'm beginning to, I can see that other people are no smarter, better looking, or competent than I am. Yes, I'm shorter than average. But I'm well within a normal range. Instead of thinking of myself as an ineffective father, I've adopted a phrase used by the child psychologist Bruno Bettelheim. He spoke of the 'good enough parent.' That's all we have to be, good enough. Not perfect. And I'm good enough. As for being a muddled teacher, I recently read the novel *Goodbye, Mr. Chips* by James Hilton. Chips started out a muddled teacher, but eventually became a highly effective one. I see now that becoming a better teacher is really a learning process, a kind of education in itself. And I'm learning."

### Anxious or Just Prudent?

Explore ways to convert anxiety into prudence.

Neurotic anxiety is characterized by excessive, irrational worry. If you have a tendency to worry, it is not likely to go away overnight by an act of will. It is a part of your neuroticism, a basic trait of your personality. However, this tendency can be given a new shape and a new name. With the use of your intelligence, the aid of the principles in this book, and the principle of compensation, you can convert anxiety into prudence. Neurotic anxiety is excessive and irrational. Prudence, however, suggests that you are careful, that you think things through, and that you look before you leap. These are all desirable traits. And they can grow from the root of anxiety. In other words, you start with the lemon of neurotic anxiety, and through a process combining experience with personal growth, you convert anxiety into the lemonade of prudence. Now you are operating at a higher, better level than people who have not had to struggle with neurotic anxiety.

You may give many of the things that you do as a neurotic person self-labels such as "overcautious" or "compulsive." Sometimes it is difficult to distinguish between being cautious and being overcautious. Some years ago I was traveling cross-country by automobile with my family. At every gas station I checked fluid levels, air pressure in my tires, and the hoses under the hood. At every stop the hoses were tight. Coming back from the East Coast, after traveling about 5,000 miles, I checked the hoses at a station in New Mexico. We were just about to cross a long stretch of desert in the middle of July. A radiator hose was loose and ready to drop off. I tightened it, and there was no problem. If I had not checked the hose, we would have had trouble right in the middle of the desert, miles from help or service. Was I compulsive or prudent? It depends on the label you want to give it. I like to think I was prudent.

Madeline H. says, "Whenever we leave the house, I have to double-check and make sure that the coffee pot is off, the iron is unplugged, the back door is locked, and so forth. I mean double-check literally. I've already checked all of these items once. But when I get to the front door, I tell my husband that I'm going to go back and double-check. He says that I'm silly, neurotic, anxious, and compulsive. On the other hand, do you know that if you do what I do, double-check everything, that two or three times a year you *will* find the back door unlocked or an appliance that is on? Maybe my neuroticism has kept the house from burning down." Is Madeline just rationalizing, making herself feel OK about being overly anxious? Or, is she prudent? Again, it depends on the label you give her behavior.

There is such a thing as neurotic anxiety. It can be a burden and excessive. However, you should not totally reject your tendency to be cautious and to worry about life. It can, within reason, be turned into a desirable trait—the trait of prudence.

Here are some ways to recognize the presence of neurotic anxiety:

- You worry even when you know that you are over-anxious or that your worry is foolish.
- Worrying excessively is interfering with the quality of your life.
- You are frequently apprehensive, thinking that something awful is going to happen even when there is no reason to think so.
- You seem to have no control over your anxiety. It controls you.
- Your fears are vague and formless.
- You frequently avoid challenging situations and opportunities because of excessive concern over things that can go wrong.
- You use phobias (i.e., irrational fears) to help you avoid things and situations that make you nervous.

A review of Chapter 15 will supply you with strategies that will help you convert anxiety into prudence.

### Depressed or Just Sensible?

**Explore ways to convert depression into a sober, sensible outlook on life.**

If you are prone to neurotic depression, it is unlikely that you will ever display the kind of sunny disposition possessed by the central character in Eleanor H. Porter's novel *Pollyanna*. In order to survive the ups and downs of life, Pollyanna invents the "glad game." She always looks on the bright side of everything.

Perhaps this is going too far. But you don't have to look on the sad side of everything either. You can compensate for your tendency toward depression, and look at life with a sober, sensible outlook that is realistic. Maybe you won't go around smiling and laughing all the time. But neither will you mope and waste your time in self-pity. A tendency toward depression is the raw psychological material that you will turn into a commonsense, realistic outlook on life.

Sloan C. is a fifty-two-year-old psychoanalyst. He says, "When I was a young man, I suffered from chronic depression. It was so severe that I seriously thought of suicide more than once. I compensated by majoring in psychology, then switching to medical school, and eventually becoming a psychoanalyst. I'm still prone to bouts of episodic mild depression, but I know how to cope with them. Most of my tendency toward depression has been converted into a somewhat solemn outlook on life. I can't say that I'm happy most of the time, but neither am I unhappy. I find my life and my work rewarding and meaningful. I know that my view of life is somewhat heavy, and I tend to look on human behavior in profound terms. Nonetheless, this is compatible with my personality. And it's a good tradeoff with depression."

Here are some ways to recognize the presence of depression:

- You are often in a low, cheerless mood.
- Your outlook on life is bleak.
- You view many situations and life tasks with a negative mental attitude.
- You seem to lack energy. And you suspect this is not because of your general health but because of your emotional disposition.
- Sometimes you move very, very slowly. You resist

going at things with enthusiasm; you feel spiritless and without drive.

- Your behavior is too often self-defeating, going against your own best long-run self-interest.
- You feel that life is a heavy burden.

A review of Chapter 16 will supply you with strategies that will help you convert depression into a sober, sensible outlook on life.

### Aggressive or Just Assertive?

❦

Explore ways to convert aggressiveness into assertiveness.

Aggressiveness, associated with neurotic anger, is a destructive trait. It is characterized by hostility toward others and sometimes by self-destructiveness. Assertiveness, on the other hand, is a desirable trait characterized by constructive accomplishment and productive channeling of aggressive tendencies.

The life of the author Jack London provides a case in point. As a young man, London was nervy and aggressive. He was an oyster pirate when he was still an adolescent. He engaged in many waterfront brawls, leading a rough and tumble life. As a young adult he became a largely self-educated person, and turned his aggressive tendencies into stories and novels that were filled with raw conflict. Two of his best-known novels, *The Call of the Wild* and *The Sea-Wolf,* are tales of struggle and survival. He went after what he wanted in life and generally got it. He was able to convert random aggressiveness into assertive accomplishment.

Margo F. is thirty-three years old, married, a mother of

two, and a high school teacher. She says, "When I was a kid, I was nasty. My mother says I was a mean child, willful and difficult to raise. And I know it's true. I was always getting into fights with my sisters and I even had a knockdown fight with another girl in high school. I once bit a boyfriend on the arm because I didn't like the way he was treating me. But little by little I learned. I grew up. I got a little bit of emotional maturity by thinking things through and reflecting on my life. I went to college, and channeled my aggressiveness into basketball. I played a forward position, and was a high scorer for the team. I majored in physical education with a minor in history. Now I teach two history classes at our high school, am a PE teacher, and coach the female basketball team. We've won our share of games and trophies. I can honestly say that my aggressive tendencies have been modified and are no longer a serious problem. I have converted them into assertiveness. Nobody pushes Margo around. But, on the other hand, I'm not hostile and I don't try to push others around."

Here are some ways to recognize the presence of neurotic anger:

- You pick verbal fights with your partner, family members, and friends for no particular reason.
- Small frustrations, frustrations that you know might not bother others much, drive you up the wall and really make you mad.
- You get very impatient when other people are talking. You wish they would be quicker and finish it; or you often interrupt them.
- You suffer from the "hurry-up sickness"—you are dissatisfied with the rate at which most events occur.
- You frequently manipulate other people or bully them.

- If you can't have your own way, even in small things, you feel your blood begin to boil.
- You are no stranger to the idea of getting mad at yourself. A little too often you think, "I could kick myself" or something similar.

A review of Chapter 17 will supply you with strategies that will help you convert aggressiveness into assertiveness.

---

### MASTER STRATEGY 19

## Look upon your neurosis as an asset, not a liability.

It is too easy to focus on all the negative aspects of being neurotic. Granted, if allowed to grow like a wild bush in your mental and emotional garden, your neurosis can result in negative effects like chronic anxiety, depression, and anger. On the other hand, by using the principle of compensation, the strategies outlined in this and prior chapters, and your intelligence, your neurosis can in fact become an asset.

Your neurosis motivates you. It is uncomfortable to suffer from emotional distress. Your efforts to overcome it will result in a learning process that brings you to higher levels than people who are free of neurosis.

As you already know, both intelligence and creativity are associated with neurosis. Research and my own observations suggest that neurotic people usually have great strengths that offset their emotional weaknesses. The overall quality of your life in terms of joy, ecstasy, or general appreciation of the special quality of life is potentially greater than your more ordinary, less imaginative companions in life—other people. Your suffering, sometimes severe, usually moderate, is the price you pay—and should be willing to pay—to enjoy the higher reaches of human experience and consciousness.

---

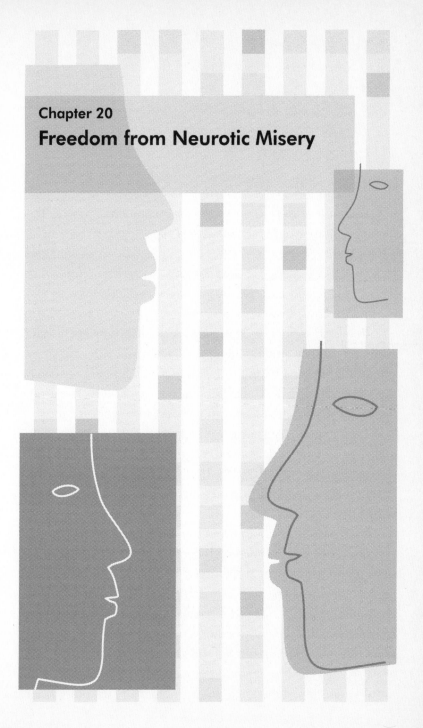

Chapter 20

# Freedom from Neurotic Misery

**Rebecca H. is one** of my psychology students. She is the divorced mother of two children and aspires to become a psychologist. She complains of frequent anxiety, depression, and lack of self-confidence. The other day, immediately following a class, she asked me, "Dr. Bruno, are you well-adjusted?"

I answered, "No."

Rebecca seemed a little surprised. "But you are a psychologist. You've studied Freud and James and Skinner. That's one of the reasons I want to become a psychologist—to help me understand myself and become well adjusted. If it's not working for you, then how can I expect it to work for me?"

I explained, "I'm not a well-adjusted person. I'm a well-adjusting person. Adjustment is a process, not an end state. It's something you have to think about all of your life. Psychology *is* working for me, but I, in turn, have to work with it."

I have on the wall in my study the framed print of an oil painting depicting a nineteenth-century clipper ship plowing through a stormy sea. It tilts over at a precarious 45-degree angle. Nonetheless, it stays afloat and makes progress. Its sails are trimmed, the vessel tacks, and it makes other adjustments to cope with the heavy weather. On sunny days with a good wind, the ship can put out full sail and place the wind directly at its stern. The ship is never permanently well adjusted. It is always adjusting, depending on the momentary circumstances.

You and I are like the sailing ship. We must learn to become adept at adjusting if we want to keep the ship of self afloat in the sea of life.

## Seven Pillars of Emotional Wisdom

To help you sail through your own stormy seas here are seven pillars of emotional wisdom. They will help you attain freedom from neurotic misery. The seven pillars are not new. You have already encountered them in various places in prior chapters. However, they encapsulate much of the earlier teachings in this book. As a consequence, I believe that you will find them to be a useful summary.

### 1. Assert Your Free Will

🍃

**You have a natural, inborn free will.**

Believing in your own free will is necessary for your mental health. It is the central pillar of emotional wisdom. It is essential that you see yourself as capable of making real choices and directing your own behavior. You must not look upon yourself as a victim of anything—genetics, fate, unhappy parenting, bad luck, or a lack of proper connections. Think of yourself as an autonomous being.

The existence or nonexistence of free will cannot be proved. Among philosophers, there is no consensus. Nonetheless, you can *affirm* your free will. If you act as if you have free will, then your behavior induces a self-fulfilling prophecy. And personal freedom will be yours. Remember that William James said, "My first act of free will was to believe in free will."

### 2. Explore Your Unconscious Motives

♥

**Being aware of your motives gives you greater self-control over your behavior.**

People are often hesitant to explore their unconscious motives. Individuals frequently see such motives as dangerous and dark—and they are. Freud compared the mind to an iceberg. Unconscious motives represent the submerged self. In the case of an actual iceberg, sonar can reveal the outlines of the hidden structure. With this knowledge, a ship can avoid concealed hazards.

Similarly, when you explore your unconscious motives, you get to know yourself—you become aware of the dangers associated with repressed, hidden impulses. When you examine your life, part of such self-examination includes taking a hard, realistic look at your unconscious motives. (Methods for self-analysis were presented in Chapters 11 and 12.)

### 3. Escape Your Bad Habits

♥

**Habits can be modified or broken.**

Bad habits often seem to have an iron grip on us. A Spanish proverb says, "Habits at first are cobwebs. Then they become cables." Yes, they are like cables that restrict our range of motion in life. They limit our choices and interfere with the execution of our free will. Irrational thoughts, adverse emotional reactions, and self-defeating behaviors are all associated with bad habits. There is no doubt that they aggravate a neurosis.

But all is not lost. Habits are learned. They are acquired through experience. They are not a part of your basic nature, only an addition to it. Consequently, there is hope. What has been learned can be unlearned. Habits can often be broken. Or, if they can't be broken completely, they can be modified to the point where they present little or no problem. (Methods for breaking and/or modifying habits were presented in Chapter 7.)

### 4. Achieve Your Potential

🔖

**Don't neglect your need to be self-actualizing.**

A self-actualizing person maximizes his or her talents and potentialities. If you don't do this, you are selling yourself short. And you will, in turn, aggravate any neurotic depression. You need to work toward becoming the person you were meant to be. You want to be sure to use whatever nature has given you in the way of special aptitudes or abilities. However, you don't have to put all of your eggs in the self-actualization basket. Sometimes an ordinary job will pay the bills, and your true calling in life can be expressed in a form that earns you little or no money. Nonetheless, such an expression is gratifying and emotionally rewarding.

### 5. Find Meaning in Life

❦

### Life can have meaning and purpose.

If your life seems to have no meaning or purpose, you are likely to suffer from an existential neurosis. This is a miserable emotional state characterized by utter demoralization. Life seems like nothing. It is pointless and absurd. This is an intolerable state of affairs from an emotional standpoint.

Fortunately, the perception that life is a sort of vacuum is an illusion. Life in fact is full of meaning and purpose. The values that give your life meaning are waiting to be discovered. And when you discover them, you will find that it is relatively easy to carry your burdens and keep walking into the future. (Ways of channeling a neurosis into a meaningful life were presented in Chapter 14.)

### 6. Embrace Your Complex Nature

❦

### Look upon your neurosis not as an affliction but as a challenge.

Yes, your neurosis has its downside. It can be the principal factor that induces chronic anxiety, depression, and anger. On the other hand, your neurosis more often than not brings with it all the assets of a complex nature—sensitivity, a powerful need for self-actualization, intelligence, and creativity. Employing your intelligence and creativity, you will discover strengths that more than offset your neurotic tendencies.

Perhaps you have the potential for more suffering than

the run-of-the-mill person. But you also have greater capacity for achievement and joy.

From time to time go back to Chapter 2 and retake the self-scoring quiz. It will give you a measure of your efforts to reduce your neurosis temperature.

### 7. Admit Your Responsibility

🔦

**Take responsibility for your own mental and emotional health.**

In your efforts to improve your mental and emotional health, you may turn to psychotherapy or to drug therapy. Either of these interventions can, under certain circumstances, be helpful. But remember that a therapist is not King Arthur's Merlin the Magician or Cinderella's Fairy Godmother. A professional has knowledge and can be helpful. But that's all. Don't expect too much. Don't idealize his or her powers and set yourself up for a crushing disappointment.

Drug therapy is not a cure for your personal problems. It is a treatment. And it can have adverse side effects. You can't just lean on a drug, making it a crutch that will take over and do the work of living for you.

In the final analysis, you have to play a significant role in recovering from the worst symptoms of a neurosis. The gains you make by your own efforts, because they require a large investment of self, are likely to be retained. Become an active participant in thinking and feeling better. It is a natural, gratifying pathway.

## MASTER STRATEGY 20

### Make the seven pillars of emotional wisdom a part of your philosophy of life.

You have a philosophy of life—stated consciously or lived unconsciously. Your philosophy of life is what you assume to be true about existence and your relationship to the world. A philosophy of life can be negative. You can believe that life is absurd, a kind of cosmic joke. This general outlook is associated with chronic anxiety, depression, and anger—the big three villains of emotional life.

Or, you can have a positive philosophy of life. You can assume that human existence is rich with meaning and purpose, that *your* life can make sense. This general outlook will help you effectively manage the villains of emotional life. If you make the seven pillars of emotional wisdom a part of your philosophy of life, you will find that they will play a constructive role in your day-to-day behavior. You can use them to think better and feel better every day.

## A Final Word

You don't have to live in neurotic misery just because you are neurotic. You can have a meaningful, rewarding life. The trick is not to "cure" yourself of your neurosis but to learn to live with it. More than that, you can, as I believe I have shown you, use your neurosis to reach heights that you might not otherwise have obtained.

And when the going gets rough, when you feel low, be sure to say quietly and firmly to yourself, "It's OK to be neurotic. I'm stronger than I think I am. I'll survive. I really will."

# Glossary

**anxiety disorder:**

A behavioral disorder characterized by chronic, irrational anxiety. The American Psychiatric Association's diagnostic manual identifies a set of such disorders. This cluster of related disorders is more or less synonymous with what most people would call a "neurosis."

**as-if world:**

We generally assume that the world we live in, including our existence and our personal future, is a solid reality. The as-if quality of the world is understood when we recognize that the world is fragile; that, for example, the future we desire may never arrive because of death or disability.

**cognitive errors:**

Tendencies to make certain persistent mistakes in the way we think. Two very common errors are *either-or thinking* and *overgeneralization*. Both are capable of intensifying anxiety.

**depression:**

A mental and emotional state characterized by a negative, pessimistic outlook on life and a low, cheerless mood. Associated signs and symptoms often include a lack of energy, a tendency to move slowly, and the conviction that life is a heavy burden.

**desensitization:**

A psychotherapeutic method of treatment characterized by repeated exposure to those things or situations that trigger anxiety. The exposure can be in life itself or in imagination. A therapist usually administers this kind of treatment; sometimes it can be effectively self-applied. With repeated exposures to fearful stimuli, the individual learns to adapt and anxiety is reduced.

**determinism:**

The point of view that we live in a cause-and-effect universe. Determinism says that you are what you are because of genetic tendencies or environmental factors. It also asserts that every thought you think, every feeling you feel, and every action you take is caused at some level.

**dream interpretation:**

A technique used in classical psychoanalysis. According to Freud, dreams, particularly those of neurotic persons, usually have two levels. The *manifest level* is what is actually dreamed. It is the story and images that are consciously remembered when one awakens. The *latent level* is what the dream means. The meaning is usually contained within a forbidden wish. The aim of dream interpretation is to reveal the meaning of the dream to the patient in order to make unconscious information available at a conscious level.

**ego defense mechanism:**

An automatic psychological mechanism that protects the ego, the conscious "I" of the personality, from reality's harsher blows. There are a group of such mechanisms, and they include denial of reality, repression, rationalization, and projection.

### ego states:

Actual states, meaning ways of thinking and acting, that your ego adopts from time to time. The three ego states are the Parent, the Adult, and the Child. These states are not to be confused with actual parents, adults, and children. When the words are capitalized, they refer to one's inner personality.

### endorphins:

Chemical messengers found in the brain. The word *endorphin* is a contraction of the two words *endogenous* and *morphine*. In other words, endorphins are natural morphine-like substances. In contrast to the abuse of illegal drugs, endorphins are generally thought of as beneficial. They help us fight pain and enhance our sense of well-being, and they definitely help us to fight depression.

### existential anxiety:

A kind of natural anxiety associated with life itself. We know that we have bodies that can and do become damaged and ill. We know that things can go wrong. Consequently, a certain amount of anxiety is built into the very fabric of existence.

### existentialism:

The point of view that life as it is actually experienced on a day-to-day basis by the individual is far more important than any so-called objective description, whether it is scientific or philosophical. According to existentialism, the experience that one has a free will is more important to the individual than an objective or scientific analysis that denies the existence of free will and stresses the importance of determinism.

**Freudian slip:**

According to Freud, an error, such as a slip of the tongue or pen, that reveals the presence of an unconscious, forbidden wish.

**genetic fatalism:**

A tendency to perceive life as controlled by your genetic tendencies, not by you as a conscious self. The biological viewpoint assumes, for example, that neuroticism is an inborn trait. If you are convinced that you are doomed to be miserable because you are neurotic, you are giving in to genetic fatalism.

**humanistic psychology:**

The point of view in psychology that human behavior has a unique quality, that it cannot be understood in terms of the behavior of animals. The broad general themes of humanistic psychology point the way toward a meaningful life. The father of humanistic psychology is Abraham Maslow.

**hysteria:**

A kind of neurotic reaction characterized by false symptoms with no real neurological basis. For example, a person may imagine that he is blind when there is nothing wrong with his eyes or optic nerves. The term *hysteria* is a classical one. In current psychiatric language, the condition is referred to as *somatoform disorder, conversion type.*

**idealization-frustration-demoralization (IFD) syndrome:**

A behavioral pattern with three distinct stages. As applied to the description of a love relationship, in the first stage of idealization, the other person is perfect or wonderful. In the second stage, if things go wrong, there is frustration. The other person doesn't act the way that you want him or her to act. In the third stage, there is demoralization. You feel burned out, fed up, and empty of joy.

### inferiority complex:

According to Alfred Adler, a set of negative interrelated ideas that one has about oneself. The ideas are not necessarily "true" in any objective sense of the word. A very bright person might see herself as unintelligent. A very attractive person might perceive himself as ugly.

### I-thou relationship:

According to theologian Martin Buber, an authentic relationship in which a first person (the "I") perceives a second person (the "thou") as a fully human individual with consciousness and feelings. A solid I-thou relationship is not manipulative and provides a foundation for emotional closeness

### learned helplessness:

A mental and emotional conditioned acquired by one or more failure experiences. The individual suffering from learned helplessness generalizes from a first situation in which he was actually helpless to a second situation in which he is not at all helpless. However, when a person suffers from learned helplessness, he acts as if he were helpless in the second situation.

### locus of control:

According to psychologist Julian Rotter, the place where you perceive the causes of your behavior to be located. If you perceive the cause of a particular behavior as arising from within the self, then this is an *internal* locus of control. If you perceive the cause of a particular behavior as arising from outside the self, then this is an *external* locus of control.

### negative practice:

As presented by psychologist Knight Dunlap, a habit-breaking method in which the individual voluntarily performs certain selected aspects of a bad habit. Dunlap referred to this as "practicing the error." Such voluntary performance of the behavior that one often fights or resists tends to undermine the strength of the habit.

### neurosis:

A condition that exists in an individual if that individual suffers chronic anxiety out of proportion to realistic threats.

### projection:

An ego defense mechanism. A projection is a perception of the external world controlled by unconscious motives. One sees others and situations in terms of one's own wishes and emotional conflicts.

### psychosis:

A pathological mental state. A psychosis exists when a person is out of touch with reality. She experiences a severe thought disorder characterized by delusions (i.e., false ideas).

### relaxation response:

According to research physician Herbert Benson, this is a natural response characterized by muscle relaxation and a reduction in anxiety. The relaxation response can be self-induced by meditation or similar techniques.

**repression:**

An ego defense mechanism characterized by a denial of inner reality. When the ego uses repression, it shoves down threatening mental and emotional information to an unconscious level. Such repressed material often includes early painful childhood memories and forbidden wishes.

**self-actualization:**

According to humanistic psychologist Abraham Maslow, an inborn tendency to maximize our talents and potentialities, to become the people nature intended us to be.

**sexual dysfunction:**

A disruption, experienced as unpleasant, in the human sexual response cycle. The four primary dysfunctions are (1) female sexual arousal disorder, (2) female orgasmic disorder, (3) premature ejaculation, and (4) male erectile disorder.

**stimulus control:**

The capacity of the individual to take control of the stimuli (i.e., sights, sounds, and aspects of a situation) that trigger an unwanted habit. This can be accomplished either by avoiding the stimuli in question or by modifying aspects of the immediate environment.

**voluntarism:**

The point of view that we have a free will. Voluntarism asserts that although we do live in a cause-and-effect universe, there are degrees of freedom in it.

# Master Strategies

### MASTER STRATEGY 1

Recognize that it really is OK to be neurotic.

### MASTER STRATEGY 2

Work to lower your neurosis temperature.

### MASTER STRATEGY 3

Adopt the positive attitude that a neurosis is
not an affliction, but a challenge.

### MASTER STRATEGY 4

Affirm that you can learn to cope effectively
with neurotic disadvantages.

### MASTER STRATEGY 5

Learn to live with your neurotic advantages so that you can
reap their harvest without paying too high a price.

### MASTER STRATEGY 6

Look upon your neurosis as something that you possess,
not as something that possesses you.

### MASTER STRATEGY 7

Accept that bad habits are acquired and
not a part of your basic personality.

### MASTER STRATEGY 8

Seek ways to convert neurotic energy
into creative accomplishments.

### MASTER STRATEGY 9

Turn your anxiety about your health
into a positive psychological asset.

### MASTER STRATEGY 10

Work toward emotional closeness with your partner.

### MASTER STRATEGY 11

Change your ego defense mechanisms from emotional
liabilities into life-enhancing assets.

### MASTER STRATEGY 12

Think about your life in psychodynamic terms.

### MASTER STRATEGY 13

Realize that we can learn to live relatively
unafraid in a world we never made.

### MASTER STRATEGY 14

Look upon your neurotic disposition as an asset, not a
liability, in your personal search for meaning.

### MASTER STRATEGY 15

Work to make a distinction between
imaginary threats and real ones.

### MASTER STRATEGY 16

Act as if you are not depressed, and it
will help your depression lift.

### MASTER STRATEGY 17

Recognize that neurotic anger is self-induced,
manufactured by your thoughts and perceptions.

### MASTER STRATEGY 18

Challenge the idea that you need psychiatric drugs.

### MASTER STRATEGY 19

Look upon your neurosis as an asset, not a liability.

### MASTER STRATEGY 20

Make the seven pillars of emotional wisdom
a part of your philosophy of life.

# Index

sexual response cycle,
133–134
excitement, 133
orgasm, 134,
plateau, 134
resolution, 134
shyness, 36
chronic, 36, 41
situational, 36
skillful will, 87
Skinner, B. F., 68, 73–74
Socrates, 159
standardized psychologist
test, 15–16
Steinbeck, John, 36
Stewart, James, 212
stimulants, 270
sugar blues, 125
superego, 49–50

**T**

Thematic Apperception Test,
259–261
thinking, 102–103
convergent, 103
divergent, 102
Tolstoy, Leo, 190
transactional analysis, 290
Twain, Mark, 85
type A behavior pattern, 255

**U**

unconditional regard, 57
unconscious level, 158–159
unconscious motives, 179, 302

**V**

valid test, 15
Valium, 3
vitamin D, 127
vitamin E, 127
voluntarism, 68–69

**W**

Watsonian slip, 179
Watson, John B., 220
willpower, 86–87
will to be, the, 109–110
will to power, 283
workaholism, 58–59
Wright, Frank Lloyd, 100

**X**

Xanax, 3